# COHORT STUDIES IN HEALTH SCIENCES

Edited by **R. Mauricio Barría**

**Cohort Studies in Health Sciences**

http://dx.doi.org/10.5772/intechopen.71243

Edited by R. Mauricio Barría

**Contributors**

Cristhian Saavedra, Muriel Ramirez-Santana, Ibrahim Janahi, Samer Hammoudeh, Wessam Gadelhaq, R. Mauricio Barría

**Notice**

Statements and opinions expressed in the chapters are these of the individual contributors and not necessarily those of the editors or publisher. No responsibility is accepted for the accuracy of information contained in the published chapters. The publisher assumes no responsibility for any damage or injury to persons or property arising out of the use of any materials, instructions, methods or ideas contained in the book.

First published in London, United Kingdom, 2018 by IntechOpen

IntechOpen is the global imprint of INTECHOPEN LIMITED, registered in England and Wales, registration number: 11086078, The Shard, 25th floor, 32 London Bridge Street

London, SE19SG – United Kingdom

Printed in Croatia

British Library Cataloguing-in-Publication Data

A catalogue record for this book is available from the British Library

Additional hard copies can be obtained from orders@intechopen.com

Cohort Studies in Health Sciences, Edited by R. Mauricio Barría

p. cm.

Print ISBN 978-1-78923-694-1

Online ISBN 978-1-78923-695-8

# Meet the editor

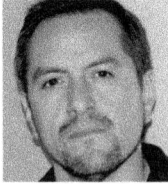

R. Mauricio Barría, DrPH, is a principal investigator and assistant professor at the Faculty of Medicine at Universidad Austral de Chile. He is currently Director of the Nursing Institute and Director of the Evidence-Based Health Office at the university. He was trained as an epidemiologist and received his MSc in Clinical Epidemiology from Universidad de la Frontera in Temuco, Chile, and his DrPH from Universidad de Chile in Santiago, Chile. His research interests lie in the areas of maternal-child health, neonatal care, and environmental health. He is skilled in epidemiological studies designs with special interest in cohort studies and clinical trials.

# Contents

**Preface IX**

Chapter 1    **Introductory Chapter: The Contribution of Cohort Studies to Health Sciences 1**
René Mauricio Barría

Chapter 2    **Prospective Cohort Studies in Medical Research 11**
Samer Hammoudeh, Wessam Gadelhaq and Ibrahim Janahi

Chapter 3    **Limitations and Biases in Cohort Studies 29**
Muriel Ramirez-Santana

Chapter 4    **Cohort Studies in the Understanding of Chronic Musculoskeletal Pain 47**
Cristhian Saavedra Santiesteban

# Chapter 1

# Introductory Chapter: The Contribution of Cohort Studies to Health Sciences

René Mauricio Barría

Additional information is available at the end of the chapter

http://dx.doi.org/10.5772/intechopen.80178

## 1. Introduction

In health sciences, the main focus is on health care using both preventive and curative actions, which are constantly evolving and being updated. In this context, research that contributes with evidence to the decision-making of health professionals is required to adequately understand health problems, as well as implement health interventions.

The fundamental aim of research in the health field is to enrich knowledge about the pathophysiological and epidemiological mechanisms of diseases and health problems and propose strategies for their prevention and treatment through different approaches and methodologies, including basic or preclinical research, clinical research, and epidemiological research in public health (**Figure 1**).

The basic or preclinical research seeks a better knowledge of the molecular, biochemical, and cellular mechanisms involved in the etiopathogenesis of diseases, forming the basis on which future studies are constructed [1]. Clinical research studies the prevention, diagnosis, and treatment of diseases along with the knowledge of their natural history that can be categorized by the period of data collection (prospective, retrospective, and transversal) as well as by its design (observational or experimental), each with its own strengths and weaknesses [2]. Finally, epidemiological research in public health and health services studies the frequency, distribution, and the health needs of the population, their risk factors, and their impact on public health [3].

In general, biomedical research consists of two main categories: in an experimental approach, the researcher deliberately exposes the subjects to a specific treatment or intervention and observes the results. These results can be compared with those obtained by a different treatment. However, in daily clinical practice, experimental studies are difficult to

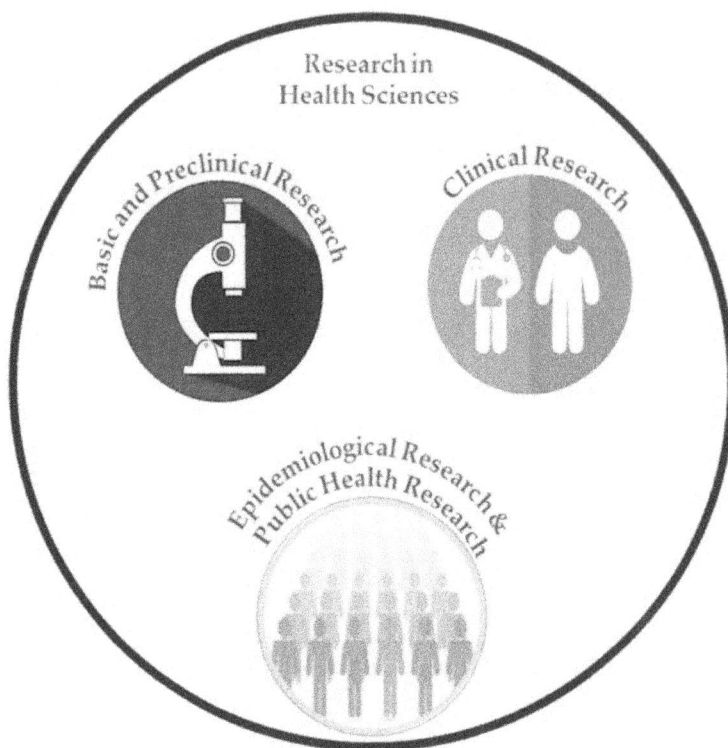

**Figure 1.** Approaches to research in health sciences.

carry out and often impose enormous logistical and budgetary challenges that are not easy to face. Therefore, health professionals can usually only observe situations and phenomena which are already segregated in groups. Therefore, researchers cannot assign an exposure or treatment, but only observe the results. This observational approach constitutes the typical environment of most clinical studies. In this context, observational studies can be classified according to the presence of a comparison group. When a comparison group is provided, the study is defined as analytical, otherwise it is considered a description. In cohort studies, the design is similar to that of clinical trials, considered the most appropriate for causal inference, with the difference that exposure occurs naturally and is determined by preferences, clinical decisions or other conditions.

As previously shown, cohorts, as well as other observational studies, have several advantages over randomized and controlled trials, including a lower cost, greater opportunity, and a wider range of patients. However, concerns about the inherent bias in these studies have limited their use when comparing treatments. Therefore, observational studies are mainly used to identify risk factors and prognostic indicators, and in situations where randomized controlled trials would be impossible or unethical [1]. Benson et al. [1] suggested that observational studies usually provide valid information and could be used to explore the available databases. Only with a greater willingness to analyze these databases would it be possible to achieve a realistic understanding of how observational studies can best be used. It should be noted that although clinical trials are considered the gold standard of clinical studies and are at the top of the traditional pyramid of scientific evidence, there may be limitations, for example, external validity that favors designs such as cohort studies [2]. Therefore, regardless of the type of research performed or evaluated in the clinical context, there must be appropriate tools to discriminate the best available evidence for health decision making [3].

## 2. General aspects of cohort studies

Cohort studies are similar to experimental studies since they are compared, exposed, and unexposed. The difference is that the researcher does not decide who is exposed, that is, does not assign the subject to one group or another; the patients go to one group to another for reasons of routine or daily clinical practice.

The word cohort means a group or group of people and has traditionally been associated with the military concept of the infantry corps of ancient Rome [4]. Consequently, the term cohort in clinical research is used to designate a group of subjects that have a characteristic, or a set of characteristics, in common (factor of study or exposure), and are followed over time [4–6]. In general, in these types of studies, a group of individuals is recruited, none of which manifests the study event at the time of recruitment, but all of which are at risk of suffering or presenting the event [5–8]. This type of study can adopt a prospective, retrospective or ambidirectional modality [4, 8–11] (**Figure 2**).

Prospective studies are planned in advance and carried out in a future period of time. The researchers pose a question and form a hypothesis about what might cause a disease and then observe a group of people over a period of time that can take several years. They collect data that may be relevant to the outcome or disease under study and, in this way, aim to detect any change in health related to the possible risk factors that they have identified.

Retrospective cohort studies examine the existing data and attempt to identify risk factors for particular conditions. For example, existing medical records are used to look back in time to identify exposed and unexposed subjects and the subsequent development (or not) of the study outcome. The study maintains the sequence from the exposure to the result, although the data collection occurred after the fact. In this case, interpretations are limited because researchers cannot go back and collect missing data.

As the name implies, in ambidirectional studies, data collection goes in both directions. This approach can be useful for exposures that have both short- and long-term results. The researcher can look back through the records that have already been collected and begin to track the subjects in the future for the onset of the outcome, or disease.

Cohorts can also be classified as closed (fixed) or open (dynamic) cohorts [5, 6, 8]. Closed or fixed cohorts (**Figure 3**) are study designs that do not consider the inclusion of a population under study beyond the recruitment period set by the researchers. That is, the participants are recruited in the same period of time and do not allow the entry of new individuals during the follow-up. All members have follow-up periods that begin at the same time.

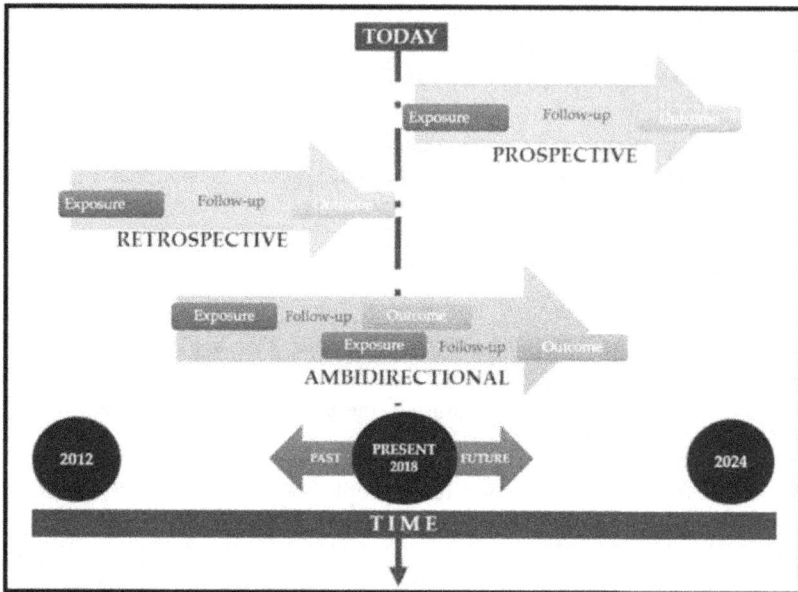

**Figure 2.** Cohort study designs.

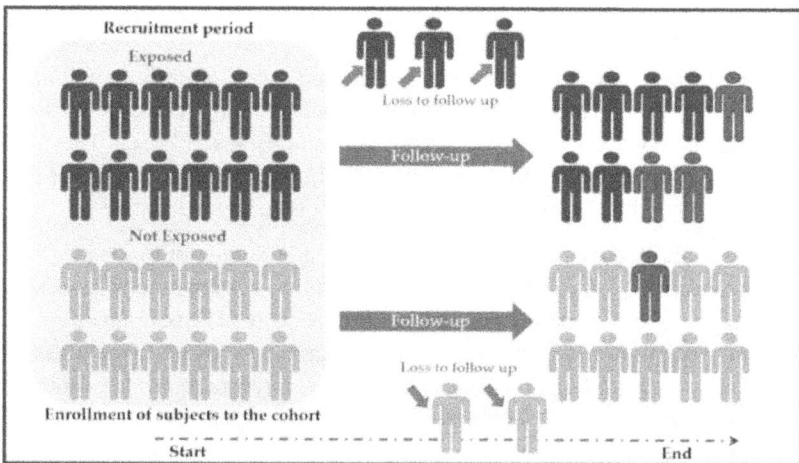

**Figure 3.** Closed (fixed) cohort study.

In contrast, in an open or dynamic cohort, individuals can enter the cohort at different times during the study period. The study allows the entry and exit of new study subjects during the follow-up phase, so the number of members may vary over time. Participants can enter or leave the cohort when they meet eligibility criteria and are often defined by geographic units and population groups (**Figure 4**).

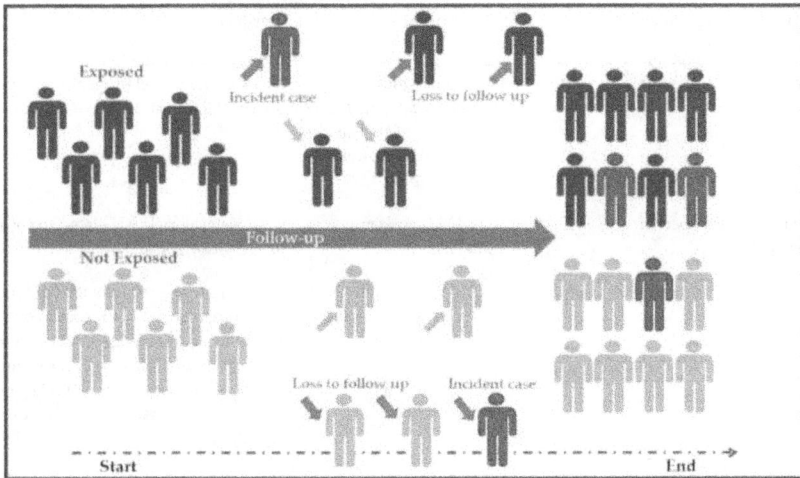

**Figure 4.** Open (dynamic) cohort study.

Some limitations should be considered when designing or analyzing a cohort study. For example, they are less suitable for studying rare diseases or diseases with a very long latency. In general, they are inadequate for identifying the causes of a sudden disease outbreak. Like any observational researches, it offers clues about the causes of the disease, rather than definitive evidence of the links between risk factors and health. Participants can leave the cohort, perhaps move away, lose contact or die from a cause that is not being studied. This can produce a bias in the results.

## 3. The contribution of cohort studies as evidence in health research

Compared with randomized controlled trials (RCTs), observational studies are likely to be faster, less expensive, and include patients that are more representative of routine clinical practice. Also, they avoid the ethical problems caused by the commitment of the therapeutic options. However, validity can be questioned by the inherent limitations of the design [12].

Analyzing the differences between the results of observational studies—such as cohort studies—and clinical trials suggests that there is little evidence of significant differences when estimating the effects between observational studies and RCTs, regardless of the study design, the heterogeneity or the inclusion of studies with pharmacological interventions. Consequently, when exploring the reasons for the lack of consistency between results from the RCTs and observational studies, other factors must be taken into account apart from the study design per se [13].

However, even with the mentioned limitations, cohort studies have delivered important findings that contribute to the understanding of multiple diseases and their risk factors (**Table 1**), for example, the Framingham Heart Study and the Nurses' Health Study, among others.

| Name of cohort study | Type of cohort study | Year | Participants | Purpose |
|---|---|---|---|---|
| Framingham heart study [14–16] | Prospective | 1948 | 5209 men and women in ages of 30–62 years residents of the eastern Massachusetts town of Framingham | To examine the relationship between several factors and cardiovascular disease |
| British doctors' cohort study [17] | Prospective | 1951 | 34,439 British male doctors | To assess the risk associated to smoking habits (lung cancer) |
| Whitehall study I [18–20] | Prospective | 1967 | 19,019 male civil service (government) employees from London, United Kingdom aged 40–69 years | To examine the role of social determinants in health; association of socioeconomic, behavioral, and metabolic characteristics with the risk of prostate cancer mortality; To assess life expectancy in relation to cardiovascular risk factors recorded in middle age |
| Nurses' health study [21, 22] | Prospective | 1976 | 121,701 female registered nurses | The primary goal of the study was to evaluate the long-term consequences of oral contraceptive (OC) use, particularly its potential association with breast cancer risk |
| Whitehall study II [23–25] | Prospective | 1986 | 10,308 (6895 men and 3413 women) civil servant aged 35–55 years | Role of social determinants of disease and mortality; to evaluate effect on health and disease of the work environment, the moderating effect on these relationships of social supports, and, the interaction between psychosocial factors in the etiology of chronic disease |
| European prospective investigation into cancer and nutrition (EPIC study) [26, 27] | Prospective | 1992 | 521,457 adults, recruited by 23 centers in 10 European countries | To examine the relationship between diet and cancer |
| The Korea nurses' health study (KNHS) [28, 29] | Prospective | 2013 | 20,213 female registered nurses aged 20–45 years from Republic of Korea | To evaluate the effects of occupational, environmental, and lifestyle risk factors on the health |
| The Dutch famine birth cohort study [30] | Retrospective | 1944/1946 | 1116 Dutch female children born I Amsterdam during the "Hunger Winter" | To examine short- and long-term effects of a limited period of extreme nutritional deprivation |
| Seveso women's health study [31, 32] | Retrospective | 1976 | Women who were newborn to 40 years of age on July 10, 1976 residing around Seveso, Italy at the time of an industrial accident on July 10, 1976 | To study the relationship of dioxin (TCDD) on reproductive health |

**Table 1.** Examples of cohort studies.

# 4. Conclusion

Cohort studies are classified as the most robust form of medical research after experiments such as randomized controlled trials and may be the only alternative for evaluating causal relationships when it is impossible to perform experimental studies. Therefore, cohorts should be considered for studying various health problems both in hospitals and in the ambulatory context.

# Conflicts of interest

The author has no conflict of interests to declare.

# Author details

René Mauricio Barría

Address all correspondence to: rbarria@uach.cl

Director of the Institute of Nursing and the Evidence-Based Health Office, Faculty of Medicine, Universidad Austral de Chile, Valdivia, Chile

# References

[1] Benson K, Hartz AJ. A comparison of observational studies and randomized, controlled trials. The New England Journal of Medicine. 2000;**342**:1878-1886. DOI: 10.1056/NEJM200006223422506

[2] Murad MH, Asi N, Alsawas M, Alahdab F. New evidence pyramid. Evidence-Based Medicine. 2016;**21**:125-127. DOI: 10.1136/ebmed-2016-110401

[3] Zeng X, Zhang Y, Kwong JS, Zhang C, Li S, Sun F, et al. The methodological quality assessment tools for preclinical and clinical studies, systematic review and meta-analysis, and clinical practice guideline: A systematic review. Journal of Evidence-Based Medicine. 2015;**8**:2-10. DOI: 10.1111/jebm.12141

[4] Grimes DA, Schulz KF. Cohort studies: Marching towards outcomes. Lancet. 2002;**359**:341-345. DOI: 10.1016/S0140-6736(02)07500-1

[5] Aschengrau A, Seage GR. Cohort studies. In: Aschengrau A, Seage GR, editors. Essentials of Epidemiology in Public Health. 3rd ed. Burlington, MA: Jones & Bartlett Learning; 2013. pp. 205-232

[6] Rothman KJ, Greenland S. Cohort studies. In: Rothman KJ, Greenland S, Lash TL, editors. Modern Epidemiology. 3rd ed. Philadelphia: Lippincott Williams & Wilkins; 2013. pp. 100-110

[7]   Sessler DI, Imrey PB. Clinical research methodology 2: Observational clinical research. Anesthesia and Analgesia. 2015;**121**:1043-1051. DOI: 10.1213/ANE.0000000000000861

[8]   Argimon J, Jiménez J. Métodos de investigación clínica y epidemiológica. 4th ed. Barcelona, España: Elsevier; 2013

[9]   Schneider D, Lilienfeld DE. Lilienfeld's Foundations of Epidemiology. 4th ed. New York: Oxford University Press; 2015

[10]  Ayres JG, Harrison RM, Nichols GL, Maynard CBERL. Environmental Medicine. London: CRC Press; 2010

[11]  Hulley SB, Cummings SR, Newman TB. Designing cross-sectional and cohort studies. In: Hulley SB, Cummings SR, Browner WS, Grady DG, Newman TB, editors. Designing Clinical Research. Philadelphia: Lippincott Williams & Wilkins; 2014. pp. 85-96

[12]  Hartz A, Bentler S, Charlton M, Lanska D, Butani Y, Soomro GM, et al. Assessing observational studies of medical treatments. Emerging Themes in Epidemiology. 2005;**2**:8. DOI: 10.1186/1742-7622-2-8

[13]  Anglemyer A, Horvath HT, Bero L. Healthcare outcomes assessed with observational study designs compared with those assessed in randomized trials. Cochrane Database of Systematic Reviews. 2014:MR000034. DOI: 10.1002/14651858.MR000034.pub2

[14]  Oppenheimer GM. Framingham heart study: The first 20 years. Progress in Cardiovascular Diseases. 2010;**53**:55-61. DOI: 10.1016/j.pcad.2010.03.003

[15]  Manson JE, Bassuk SS. The Framingham offspring study—A pioneering investigation into familial aggregation of cardiovascular risk. American Journal of Epidemiology. 2017;**185**:1103-1108. DOI: 10.1093/aje/kwx068

[16]  Bitton A, Gaziano TA. The Framingham heart study's impact on global risk assessment. Progress in Cardiovascular Diseases. 2010;**53**:68-78. DOI: 10.1016/j.pcad.2010.04.001

[17]  Doll R, Peto R, Wheatley K, Gray R, Sutherland I. Mortality in relation to smoking: 40 years' observations on male British doctors. BMJ. 1994;**309**:901-911. DOI: 10.1136/bmj.309.6959.901

[18]  Batty GD, Jokela M, Kivimaki M, Shipley M. Examining the long-term association of personality with cause-specific mortality in London: Four decades of mortality surveillance in the original Whitehall smoking cessation trial. American Journal of Epidemiology. 2016;**184**:436-441. DOI: 10.1093/aje/kwv454

[19]  Batty GD, Kivimaki M, Clarke R, Davey SG, Shipley MJ. Modifiable risk factors for prostate cancer mortality in London: 40 years of follow-up in the Whitehall study. Cancer Causes & Control. 2011;**22**:311-318. DOI: 10.1007/s10552-010-9691-6

[20]  Clarke R, Emberson J, Fletcher A, Breeze E, Marmot M, Shipley MJ. Life expectancy in relation to cardiovascular risk factors: 38 year follow-up of 19,000 men in the Whitehall study. BMJ. 2009;**339**:b3513. DOI: 10.1136/bmj.b3513

[21]  Rice MS, Eliassen AH, Hankinson SE, Lenart EB, Willett WC, Tamimi RM. Breast cancer research in the nurses' health studies: Exposures across the life course. American Journal of Public Health. 2016;**106**:1592-1598. DOI: 10.2105/AJPH.2016.303325

We are IntechOpen,
the world's leading publisher of
Open Access books
Built by scientists, for scientists

**3,750+**
Open access books available

**115,000+**
International authors and editors

**119M+**
Downloads

Our authors are among the

**151**
Countries delivered to

**Top 1%**
most cited scientists

**12.2%**
Contributors from top 500 universities

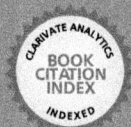

Interested in publishing with us?
Contact book.department@intechopen.com

Numbers displayed above are based on latest data collected.
For more information visit www.intechopen.com

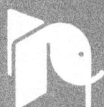

[22] Colditz GA. Nurses' health study: Demonstrating the impact of research, and adapting new measures and approaches to increase relevance and effect of cohort studies. Public Health Research and Practice. 2016;26:2631628. DOI: 10.17061/phrp2631628

[23] Marmot M, Brunner E. Cohort profile: The Whitehall II study. International Journal of Epidemiology. 2005;34:251-256. DOI: 10.1093/ije/dyh372

[24] Brunner EJ, Shipley MJ, Ahmadi-Abhari S, Valencia HC, Abell JG, Singh-Manoux A, et al. Midlife contributors to socioeconomic differences in frailty during later life: A prospective cohort study. The Lancet Public Health. 2018;3:e313-e322. DOI: 10.1016/S2468-2667(18)30079-3

[25] Xue B, Cadar D, Fleischmann M, Stansfeld S, Carr E, Kivimaki M, et al. Effect of retirement on cognitive function: The Whitehall II cohort study. European Journal of Epidemiology. 2017. DOI: 10.1007/s10654-017-0347-7. In press

[26] Gonzalez CA, Pera G, Agudo A, Bueno-de-Mesquita HB, Ceroti M, Boeing H, et al. Fruit and vegetable intake and the risk of stomach and oesophagus adenocarcinoma in the European prospective investigation into cancer and nutrition (EPIC-EURGAST). International Journal of Cancer. 2006;118:2559-2566. DOI: 10.1002/ijc.21678

[27] van Veldhoven CM, Khan AE, Teucher B, Rohrmann S, Raaschou-Nielsen O, Tjonneland A, et al. Physical activity and lymphoid neoplasms in the European prospective investigation into cancer and nutrition (EPIC). European Journal of Cancer. 2011;47:748-760. DOI: 10.1016/j.ejca.2010.11.010

[28] Kim O, Ahn Y, Lee HY, Jang HJ, Kim S, Lee JE, et al. The Korea nurses' health study: A prospective cohort study. Journal of Women's Health (2002). 2017;26:892-899. DOI: 10.1089/jwh.2016.6048

[29] Lee JE, Song S, Cho E, Jang HJ, Jung H, Lee HY, et al. Weight change and risk of uterine leiomyomas: Korea nurses' health study. Current Medical Research and Opinion. 2018:1-7. DOI: 10.1080/03007995.2018.1462783. In press

[30] Lumey LH, Ravelli AC, Wiessing LG, Koppe JG, Treffers PE, Stein ZA. The Dutch famine birth cohort study: Design, validation of exposure, and selected characteristics of subjects after 43 years follow-up. Paediatric and Perinatal Epidemiology. 1993;7:354-367. DOI: 10.1111/j.1365-3016.1993.tb00415.x

[31] Ames J, Warner M, Brambilla P, Mocarelli P, Satariano WA, Eskenazi B. Neurocognitive and physical functioning in the Seveso women's health study. Environmental Research. 2018;162:55-62. DOI: 10.1016/j.envres.2017.12.005

[32] Eskenazi B, Mocarelli P, Warner M, Samuels S, Vercellini P, Olive D, et al. Seveso women's health study: A study of the effects of 2,3,7,8-tetrachlorodibenzo-p-dioxin on reproductive health. Chemosphere. 2000;40:1247-1253. DOI: 10.1016/S0045-6535(99)00376-8

# Prospective Cohort Studies in Medical Research

Samer Hammoudeh, Wessam Gadelhaq and
Ibrahim Janahi

Additional information is available at the end of the chapter

http://dx.doi.org/10.5772/intechopen.76514

## Abstract

Cohort studies are the analytical design of observational studies that are epidemiologically used to identify and quantify the relationship between exposure and outcome. Due to the longitudinal design, cohort studies have several advantages over other types of observational studies. The purpose of this chapter is to cover the various characteristics of prospective cohort studies. This chapter is divided into three main sections. In the first we introduce the concept and ranking of cohort studies, as well as the advantages and disadvantages. In the second we focus on the design of cohort studies, mainly its prospective aspect, and the distinguishing features from the retrospective type. The section also covers the essential characteristics of a cohort study design and its varied applications in medical research. In the third we go over examples of prospective studies in the medical field. For each, an overview of the study design is given, along with a random selection of study findings/impact, strengths and weaknesses.

**Keywords:** observational study, cohort study, prospective cohort study, longitudinal study, study design, epidemiology, medical research

# 1. Cohort studies

## 1.1. Introduction

The term "cohort" originates from Latin "cohors" [1]. A term that was used in the military back in Roman times, which referred to a unit that is comprised of 300–600 men, of which each 10 cohorts were named a legion [2]. In the field of epidemiology, Frost was the first to introduce the term "cohort study" back in 1935 [3]. Cohort refers to a group of individuals that share a common factor or a defining characteristic [4, 5], or in other words, cohort is a certain component of a specific population that can be measured and followed throughout time [6]. Cohort studies are classified under the non-experimental type of studies [4], which are observational by default [7].

A cohort study follows people as groups, two or more, from exposure to outcome [2, 8]. The two groups would be categorized based on their exposure status to "exposed" and "unexposed" [4, 9, 10]. If there were multiple groups then these would be categorized either by the type or level of exposure [4]. The main characteristic of a cohort study is that it follows participants in a forward manner, from the presence of the exposure to the presence of the outcome [2, 9–11]. Or as De Rango describes it: using a longitudinal pattern, a cohort study, follows a group or groups of individuals over time in order to ascertain the incidence of a predetermined outcome after being exposed to a certain factor, whether being a risk factor, medication, or intervention [12]. Cohort studies can either be prospective (concurrent) or retrospective (non-concurrent) [9].

### 1.2. Ranking of cohort studies

Researchers agree that cohort studies, as related to the hierarchy of evidence, rank below meta-analysis, systematic review and randomized controlled trial, but rank higher than case–control studies, cross sectional studies, case series/reports [13–16]. As newer models or classifications of the hierarchy of evidence have emerged, where meta-analysis and systematic reviews have been removed from the hierarchy and repositioned as a magnifying glass or a lens through which evidence from other types of studies can be viewed or scrutinized; cohort studies remain below randomized controlled trials and higher than the other types [17]. Cohort studies provide information on the relationship between exposure and outcome when a randomized controlled trial is not possible to conduct for whatever reason [6, 15].

### 1.3. Advantages of cohort studies

Cohort studies are the design of choice when randomization is not practical or ethical [6, 18]. They are also useful in the study of infections [9] and for hypothesis generation [19]. Due to the design of cohort studies, and since temporal sequence is present, both incidence rate and cumulative incidence can be calculated [2, 8, 20–22]. They also allow for the measurement of relative risk (RR) [2, 8, 23], hazard ratio [8], and attributable risk [8, 23]. Furthermore, they allow for the study of multiple outcomes that can be associated with a single type of exposure [2, 20] or multiple exposures [18]. Additionally, they allow for the study of rare exposures [2, 18, 20]. Finally, cohort studies have lower risk of encountering survivor bias [2], and recall bias [9, 21]. Survivor bias occurs when focusing only on those who survived or made it through a certain criteria or point, and ignoring those that didn't, such as studying rapidly fatal diseases [2].

### 1.4. Disadvantages of cohort studies

Among the disadvantages of cohort studies is selection bias, which may occur when the participants are not representative of the population or of the patient grouping that they fall under. This in turn will influence how well or not the results can be generalized to the rest of the population, in what is known as external validity [2, 12, 18, 24, 25]. This will be covered later in section three of this chapter under aspects of cohort studies. Another disadvantage is that causation cannot be established from cohort studies [18, 20], as it would require an experimental design in order to determine any causal effect [20]. However, due to the longitudinal design of cohort studies, they may aid in studying a certain causal hypothesis [20]. A third disadvantage is that they require a large sample size, which might pose an issue when dealing with outcomes that take a long time to develop [10]. Finally, cohort studies cannot be used to study rare outcomes [23].

## 2. Prospective cohort studies

### 2.1. Types of cohort studies

Cohort studies are either prospective or retrospective [1, 2, 18]. In the former, the researcher would assess exposure at baseline and then follow the person over time in order to determine the outcome such as the development of a disease [9, 18, 20, 21, 26]. In the latter, the order is reversed, as a cohort is established after the follow up has been conducted, or the outcome has developed, and exposure is then assessed in a retrospective manner [9, 18, 20, 21, 27]. Merrill indicates that the outcome status at the start of the study is what determines the overall study type. If the outcome has not yet developed then it is a prospective study, and if the outcome has already developed then it is a retrospective study [23]. Cohort studies can also be classified based on whether or not participants are replaced once they are lost. If those that drop out or are lost to follow up are replaced with new participants, then this would be classified as a dynamic or an open cohort. In the case that those lost do not get replaced, then it would be classified as a fixed or closed cohort [4, 20].

#### 2.1.1. Prospective cohort studies

Prospective cohort studies, as the name indicates, observes a group of people after being exposed to a certain factor in order to investigate the outcome, following the natural sequence of time, starting with the present and looking forward in time [12, 18, 20], which in turn provides true risk (absolute) estimates for the groups under investigation [26]. It is considered the gold standard among observational studies [8]. Under this type of study, the researcher would have control over data collection methodology, as well as the overall cohort study set up, which gives prospective cohort studies an advantage over retrospective cohort studies [9]. Further advantages and disadvantages of prospective cohort studies are discussed below.

##### 2.1.1.1. Advantages of prospective cohort studies

Euser et al. highlight the major advantage of prospective cohort studies as being accurate in regards to the information collected about exposures, endpoints, and confounders [18]. Others list the following as advantages of prospective cohort studies; first: the exposure has already been measured before the outcome has occurred, which allows for the assessment of temporal sequence [28]. This allows for the calculation of incidence and the determination of the disease process [2, 12, 20, 23]. Second: elimination of recall bias, as there is no need for any recollection of information since the data is being collected in a prospective manner [7]. However, Kip et al. reported that recall bias can pose an issue in prospective cohort studies if the exposure is self-reported, brief, and requires multiple measurements, such as stress episodes [29]. Third: It allows for the study of exposures were randomization is not practical or ethical [12]. Fourth: it allows for the study of rare exposures [20]. Fifth: it allows for the study of multiple outcomes [20, 26].

### 2.1.1.2. Disadvantages of prospective cohort studies

Among the disadvantages of prospective cohort studies is the loss to follow up, which is common among cohort studies. This can ultimately lead to differential loss to follow up among those exposed and unexposed, which in turn can complicate the interpretation of the results [2, 7, 12, 18, 24]. Another disadvantage is that they are time consuming if follow up periods are far apart. This would be resource consuming as well, which would make prospective cohort studies not suitable for the study of outcomes that take long time to develop [18, 20, 24, 26]. A third disadvantage is that they are expensive to conduct [18, 20, 30]. The third section of this chapter is dedicated to providing examples of prospective cohort studies.

### 2.1.2. Retrospective cohort studies

As previously described, retrospective cohort studies, also known as historic [28] or historical [24] cohorts, use data that has already been collected, such as databases of healthcare records, in order to investigate the association between the exposure and the outcome [22, 24, 26, 28]. Although the outcome has already occurred, the design of retrospective cohort studies is similar to those of prospective cohort studies [22]. They also have similar advantages and disadvantages [26, 28]. Hess indicates that retrospective studies in general are useful as pilot studies for future prospective studies [31].

Retrospective cohort studies have advantages and disadvantages. They are time efficient and cheap since the data has been collected previously and is available for scrutiny [18, 20, 26]. Additionally, since the exposure has already been measured before the outcome has occurred, this allows for the assessment of temporal sequence [28]. However, retrospective cohort studies use information that has been collected in the past for another objective other than the current study [18], and in some cases, collected for a purpose that is not related to medical research [9]. Due to this factor, the investigator lacks control over the collection of data [24, 26, 27]. Additionally, the measurement of exposure and outcome might be inconsistent or inaccurate, which can become a source of bias [24, 27, 28, 31, 32].

Examples of retrospective cohort studies:

> High plasma phosphate as a risk factor for decline in renal function and mortality in pre-dialysis patients [18, 33]. In this study, Voormolen et al. followed the clinical course among incident pre-dialysis patients, using medical charts, to study the decline in kidney function and its association with plasma phosphate levels [18, 33].

Assessment of female sex as a risk factor in atrial fibrillation in Sweden: nationwide retrospective cohort study [28, 34]. In this study, Friberg et al. investigated gender differences in the incidence of stroke among those with atrial fibrillation using the Swedish hospital discharge registry [28, 34].

Outcomes of care by hospitalists, general Internists, and family physicians [35]. In this study, Lindenauer et al. collected data from various hospitals in the USA, and compared the outcome of patients treated by the three types of care provider [35].

### 2.1.3. Aspects of cohort studies

#### 2.1.3.1. Validity

Validity is the epidemiological assessment to the lack of systematic error [4, 11]. There are two types of validity: internal validity and external validity [4, 11, 25]. *Internal validity* refers to the inferences made from the study that are related to the same source population [4, 5, 11, 25, 36], as to whether or not the study has measured what it had originally planned on measuring [25, 36]. For an example, if the exposure caused the observed change in the outcome, then the study would be considered to have high internal validity [11]. On the other hand, if the observed change in the outcome was caused by a systematic error (bias), then the study would be considered to have low internal validity [11]. Threats or violations to internal validity will be discussed later in this section under bias.

*External validity* refers to the degree to which the study results can be generalized to other populations [4, 5, 11, 25, 36]. For example, if the study participants were not representative of the general population, then the study results cannot be generalizable to others [12]. The highest level of external validity occurs when the results can be generalized to three other domains: other populations, other environments, and other times [36]. External validity can be improved by using random selection [37].

It is essential to have internal validity in order to establish external validity; that is the study must have internal validity in the first place in order to have external validity [4, 11]. For an example, if the exposure caused the observed change in the outcome, then the results can be generalizable to others. If the observed change was caused by any other factor, then the results cannot be generalized to others [4, 11]. Based on the validity hierarchy, cohort studies are considered to have low internal validity, while the external validity is high [11, 16].

#### 2.1.3.2. Bias

Bias is a study systematic error in the design, conduct, or analysis that can be categorized into three main categories: selection bias, information bias, and confounding [4, 25, 38]. *Selection bias* occurs when the sample chosen for the study is not obtained randomly, so that the sample chosen is no longer representative of the overall population [4, 25, 38, 39]. This type of bias includes three types: attrition bias, non-respondent bias, and the healthy entrant effect [38]. Attrition bias, or loss to follow up bias, occurs due to dropouts or death, which can be encountered in studies with long follow up durations (prospective) [23]. Non-respondent bias occurs when those that respond are different than those that don't respond. For example, nonsmokers are more likely to return questionnaires about smoking than smokers are [25]. The healthy entrant effect or the healthy worker effect occurs when there are differences between those that are exposed and those that are not exposed. For an example, when comparing working individuals to the general population, as workers are more likely to be healthier than the general population. In order to avoid this type of bias, it is recommended to use two similar groups, such as using two groups of working individuals [23].

*Information bias* (measurement bias) [25], occurs when the data obtained is being recorded inaccurately [4, 25, 38–40]. This type of bias can be differential (nonrandom) or nondifferential (random) as related to the outcome [4, 9, 23, 25]. The former is dependent on other variables and leads to overestimation or underestimation of any possible association, while the latter is independent from other variables and leads to underestimation of any possible association [4, 9, 23], and if the exposure was dichotomous, this type leads to bias towards the null [9]. Non differential is more commonly encountered in cohort studies [9]. Information bias can be reduced by using standardized assessment tools that have been validated [9]. Information bias is also known as classification bias, observation bias [25], or misclassification bias [23].

*Confounding:* confounding is a distortion of the effect [4, 25] that may lead to overestimation or underestimation of an effect, or even reversing the direction of an effect [4]. A confounding factor is a risk factor that is associated with the exposure and influences the outcome, however, is not related to the causation sequence [4, 25, 39]. Unlike selection and information bias, confounding can be controlled for prior to study initiation, or after study completion [25]. Controlling for confounding factors can be accomplished through: restriction, matching, stratification, and using multivariate techniques [23, 25, 27].

Restriction would involve excluding those with the confounding factor [23, 25]. If the confounding factor is categorical, then participants that fall within that category would be excluded [4], such as if smoking was considered to be a confounding factor, then those that smoke would be excluded [25]. If the confounding factor was continuous, such as age, then a range of that variable would be used to restrict the confounding [4]. Matching would involve choosing two groups that are similar to each other as much as possible [23, 25, 41], such as matching by gender or age [39]. Matching can be either individual matching or frequency matching. The former involves matching on an individual participant level, while the latter refers to matching on a group level [4]. Overmatching may occur when matching is being used, which may reflect on the statistical efficiency, validity, or cost efficiency of the study [4]. After the completion of the study, and during the analysis stage, stratification can be used to control for confounding by dividing the groups into several subgroups that are based on the confounding factor [23, 25, 39, 41]. Multivariate techniques are also used during the analysis stage and allow for the control of multiple factors [25, 39, 41].

### 2.1.3.3. Exposure and risk

Exposure must be determined using a clear and accurate definition [2, 22], which in some cases may involve levels of exposure [2]. This helps in eliminating possible selection bias [2]. The challenge becomes greater when there are multiple exposure assessments over an extended period of time [30]. The validity and the cost are two important aspects that must be taken into consideration when selecting an exposure measurement tool [30].

Both groups, those exposed and those that are not exposed should be at risk of eventually developing the outcome at some stage [2]. The exclusion criteria should exclude those that are not at risk of developing the outcome [24]. For an example, a study investigating the role of antipsychotics in the development of diabetes, should exclude those with diabetes to start with, since they are not at risk [10]. This helps in eliminating possible selection bias [2].

### 2.1.3.4. Outcomes

Outcomes should have a clear and specific definition from the beginning of the study [2, 22], which must be measurable as well [2, 22]. Outcomes should also be measured in a similar manner across all participants [2, 22]. This helps in eliminating possible information bias [2]. It is recommended to use measurement tools that have been previously validated when dealing with secondary data, and to blind those who are assessing the outcome when dealing with primary data [10].

### 2.1.3.5. Controls

The comparison group or controls (unexposed group) should be similar to the exposed group in all possible aspects, but differ in regards to the exposure itself [2]. Three types of controls can be used, with the first being the most preferable: internal comparisons, other external cohorts, and the general population [2].

### 2.1.3.6. Follow up

To avoid loss to follow up and its consequent effects on the validity of the study results; measures should be taken in order to minimize the attrition rate [2, 22, 24, 27, 42]. Some of these actions include excluding those that are at high risk of not committing to the study, providing incentives for participation, collecting personal information that would allow or facilitate future contact, and maintaining ongoing contact on regular basis during the conduction period of the study [2, 23, 24, 27]. The maximum acceptable limit for loss to follow up is 20% [23, 24, 42].

### 2.1.3.7. Precision

Precision is based on the absence of random error or chance [4, 11]. This random variation can be due to the sample itself, or how it was selected, or how it was measured [4, 11]. Standard deviations and confidence intervals are useful in determining the precision of a study, as a large standard deviation or a wide confidence interval would indicate low precision [11]. Random error or variation can be reduced by increasing the sample size [4, 27, 43], improving how you sample and how you measure, in addition to using the appropriate statistical methods [43].

### 2.1.3.8. Analysis of data

The main statistical term or product of cohort studies is the relative risk or risk ratio [6, 21], which represents the risk of developing the outcome among those that are exposed in relation to those that are not exposed [20]. An RR that is equivalent to 1 indicates an absence of any type of association. An RR that is greater than 1 would indicate that there is a positive correlation between the exposure and risk of developing a disease. An RR that is smaller than 1 would indicate the presence of a protective effect between the exposure and the outcome [12]. Other outcome measures include: hazard ratios, survival curves, and life-table rates [2]. Some of the common statistical analysis involving cohort studies include: analysis of variance (ANOVA), multivariate analysis of variance (MANOVA), mixed effect regression model, and generalized estimating equation models [7].

### 2.1.3.9. Reporting

The reporting of prospective cohort studies should follow the STROBE guidelines [12], which also apply to other observational studies [41, 44]. This acronym stands for: Strengthening the Reporting of Observational Studies in Epidemiology. These guidelines were designed by a group of international scholars including journal editors, epidemiologists, statisticians and researchers in order to set universal standards when reporting observational studies. It is comprised of a 22 item checklist that precisely dictates what should be reported under each section of an article [44–47]. Sessler and Imrey indicate that the most crucial ones are related to the study: objectives, methodology, definitions, source of data, statistical analysis, participants, and results [41]. Further information can be found at http://www.strobe-statement.org/.

Bookwala et al. outlined three main factors that aid in evaluating prospective cohort studies in their article titled "the three-minute appraisal of a prospective cohort study". These are related to (1) comparison groups selection; (2) the impact of confounding variables; (3) type of analytical strategy used [48]. Finally, the equator network (which is supported by the University of Oxford, UK, and aims to improve the quality and transparency of health research) provides guidelines and instructions for the reporting of various kinds of studies. These can be found at www.equator-network.org. Additional information regarding what to look for in a cohort study, as well as evaluation checklists can be found elsewhere [2, 8, 11, 25, 39, 48, 49]. The next section of this chapter will cover examples of famous prospective cohort studies from the medical field.

# 3. Examples of prospective cohort studies

## 3.1. The Framingham Heart Study

### 3.1.1. Overview

The Framingham heart study, initiated in 1948 by The National Heart Institute (currently the National Heart, Lung, and Blood Institute) [50], is considered to be the longest, ongoing, prospective cohort study in the history of the USA [51]. Others view it as a live model that illustrates the cohort design [52]. The study was based on the hypothesis that arteriosclerosis and hypertensive cardiovascular disease are the result of several causation factors combined rather than an individual factor [53]. Based on this, the aim of the study was to investigate the factors that contribute to the development of cardiovascular disease (CVD) by following a large cohort of individuals over a long period of time [50]. Back then in 1951, when the first article about the study was published, little was known about arteriosclerosis and hypertensive cardiovascular disease [53].

The original cohort included 5209 participants, ages 30–62 years, that were recruited at the beginning of the study in the town of Framingham, Massachusetts, USA [50]. The same cohort has been followed since initiation every two years for physical, laboratory, and lifestyle examinations [50]. The second generation, the offspring cohort, was recruited in 1971 and included 5124 participants. While 1994 witnessed the enrollment of the first Omni cohort (n = 506), in order to diversify the study population. More recently in 2002, the third generation cohort (n = 4095) was enrolled, while in 2003 the new offspring cohort (n = 103), and the second Omni group (n = 410) was enrolled [50]. The study continues to follow these cohorts every 2–6 years [54]. This multi generation, multi ethnicity, enrollment design aided significantly in the study of genetics in relation to a wide range of factors and illnesses [51, 54].

Based on the Framingham study data, since initiation and through November 2017, a total of 3561 articles have been published so far [55]. The accumulation of knowledge that has risen from this study has shed the light on cardiovascular disease risk factors [50, 51, 56], by further expanding on our understanding of chronic illnesses such as diabetes, obesity, metabolic syndrome and nonalcoholic fatty liver disease [51, 57]. Such risk factors include high blood pressure, high cholesterol levels, smoking, obesity, diabetes, and physical inactivity [50, 57].

The study was the basis of which the Framingham risk score was built on [56]. Initially published by Wilson et al. in 1998 [58], it allows for the calculation of a 10 year risk estimate of developing coronary heart disease (CHD) based on the levels of different variables [56, 58]. This would allow for the undertaking of preventive measures [56]. Later on in 2002, the Adult Treatment Panel of the National Cholesterol Education Program used the risk score as a foundation for its risk calculator [56].

### 3.1.2. Study findings

The study website (https://www.framinghamheartstudy.org/about-fhs/research-milestones. php) covers a long list of findings, among those; cigarette smoking was discovered to increase ones risk of developing heart disease back in 1960. In 1970, high blood pressure was discovered to increase ones risk of stroke. In 1988, the beneficial effects of HDL cholesterol were discovered. In 2002, the study found that obesity is considered a risk factor leading to heart failure. More recently in 2010 sleep apnea was linked to a higher risk of stroke [59]. More information and a full list of research milestones can be found elsewhere [59].

### 3.1.3. Strengths and weaknesses

In addition to what had been previously discussed regarding the benefits of the prospective design of the study, a high retention rate is among the strengths of the Framingham Heart Study as participants continue to return for their follow up visits despite the years [54].

Among the weaknesses is that the study was conducted in one population residing in one locality [7], which in turn reflects on the ability to generalize findings to other populations [58]. Another weakness is that the study cohort was not randomly selected, as investigators had to use volunteers in order to obtain the necessary sample. The final cohort ended up being more healthy when compared to the general population [7, 60].

### 3.2. The Nurses' Health Study (NHS)

#### 3.2.1. Overview

This National Institutes of Health (NIH) funded study started in 1976 [61], and as of today includes more than 275,000 participants and counting, as the Nurses' Health Study 3 is still recruiting subjects [62]. The study looks into the risk factors that have been implicated in major chronic diseases among women [62]. Initially, the study focused on heart disease, cancer, smoking, and contraceptive methods [61]. As the study evolved, it investigated many other lifestyle factors, characteristics, and diseases [61, 63].

The original cohort of the study has been followed up on by mail every two years, with a minimum response rate of 90% [61]. The second cohort, under NHS 2, was enrolled in 1989 and included 116,430 women. These also were followed up on using mail every two years. A food frequency questionnaire was added in 1991 and was mailed out every four years, with a response rate of 85–90%. Later on blood and urine samples were collected from participants [61]. The third cohort, under NHS 3, was enrolled in 2010 and is still enrolling, with a goal of diversifying the study population to include other ethnic backgrounds [61].

#### 3.2.2. Study findings

The study website (http://www.nurseshealthstudy.org/about-nhs/key-contributions-scientific-knowledge) covers numerous study findings, such as reporting lower risk of colon cancer and polyps with higher levels of vitamin D [64]. Also among the findings, Giovannucci et al. reported lower risk rates of colon cancer with longer duration of aspirin usage [65]. Baer et al. reported on mortality related risk factors among the NHS cohort [66]. Other findings related to breast cancer, CHD, stroke, colon cancer, hip fracture, cognitive function, and eye disease, in relation to cigarette smoking, oral contraceptives, post-menopausal hormone therapy obesity, alcohol, and diet can be found elsewhere [64, 67–79]. More recently Colditz et al. summarized the findings and impact of the three NHS studies in an article published in the American Journal of Public Health [80].

#### 3.2.3. Strengths and weaknesses

With focus on women, it is considered to be the longest and largest running prospective cohort study that investigates the role of lifestyle on health [63]. Among the strengths of this study is that it included multiple assessments of the various lifestyle characteristics and exposure factors [63, 80], in turn, it also contributed to the methodology of lifestyle assessment in general, which has been used in other studies [63, 80]. Additionally, it allowed for the calculation of mortality rates [63]. As for the weaknesses, white women dominated the original cohort, which reflects on the generalizability of the study results [4, 63].

### 3.3. The Caerphilly Prospective Study (CAPS)

*3.3.1. Overview*

Also known as the Caerphilly Heart Disease Study, this study was conducted in Caerphilly, South Wales, UK, and focused on ischemic heart disease (IHD) in relation to hormones, hemostatic factors, and lipids [81]. As the study evolved, other investigations were included which looked into cognitive function, stroke and hearing problems [81].

The study included four phases. In the first phase, 2512 males, ages 45–59 years, were recruited in 1979. The procedures included blood tests, electrocardiogram (ECG), clinical history, lifestyle and IHD related questionnaires [81]. The second phase ran from 1984 to 1988 and included 447 males. An audiometry test was added to the list of investigations that were included in the first phase [81]. Phase 3 took place from 1989 to 1993 and added a cognitive function test and a bleeding time test [81]. Phase 4 was conducted from 1993 to 1997, which included the audiometry and cognitive function tests originally included in the second and third phases, respectively [81]. Follow up was conducted at a later stage through mail. The study has accumulated in a total of 150 studies and counting [81].

*3.3.2. Study findings*

Among the findings of the Caerphilly Prospective study; Elwood et al. showed that adopting a healthy lifestyle was associated with lower rates of chronic disease, as well as less cognitive impairment and dementia [82]. In other findings, Mertens et al. reported an inverse association between CVD and adopting a healthy diet [83], while Bolton et al. reported an inverse association between mid-life lung function and arterial stiffness among men [84]. Additional findings can be found elsewhere [85–91].

### 3.4. Conclusion

The three sections of this chapter covered the two types of cohort studies. Observational studies in general and cohort studies in specific are a good source of information when an experiment is not feasible. Prospective cohort studies provide valuable information when studying the relationship between exposure and outcome. As with any type of study, prospective cohort studies come with advantages and disadvantages that need to be taken into consideration when interpreting the results of these studies.

## Conflict of interest

The author(s) declare no conflict of interest.

## Abbreviations

| | |
|---|---|
| ANOVA | analysis of variance |
| CAPS | Caerphilly Prospective Study |
| CVD | cardiovascular disease |
| CHD | coronary heart disease |
| ECG | electrocardiogram |
| IHD | ischemic heart disease |
| RR | relative risk |
| MANOVA | multivariate analysis of variance |
| NHS | Nurses' Health Study |
| NIH | National Institutes of Health |

## Author details

Samer Hammoudeh, Wessam Gadelhaq and Ibrahim Janahi*

*Address all correspondence to: ijanahi@hamad.qa

Hamad Medical Corporation, Doha, Qatar

## References

[1] Morabia A. A History of Epidemiologic Methods and Concepts. Birkhäuser: Switzerland, Basel; 2004

[2] Grimes DA, Schulz KF. Cohort studies: Marching towards outcomes. The Lancet. 2002; **359**(9303):341-345

[3] Doll R. Cohort studies: History of the method. I. Prospective cohort studies. Sozial- und Praventivmedizin. 2001;**46**(2):75-86

[4] Rothman KJ, Greenland S, Lash TL. Modern Epidemiology. 3rd ed. Philadelphia: Wolters Kluwer Health/Lippincott Williams & Wilkins, c2008; 2008

[5] Bryman A. Social research methods. 4th ed. Oxford; New York: Oxford University Press; 2012

[6] Mann CJ. Observational research methods. Research design II: Cohort, cross sectional, and case-control studies. Emergency Medicine Journal. 2003;**20**(1):54

[7]   Caruana EJ, Roman M, Hernández-Sánchez J, Solli P. Longitudinal studies. Journal of Thoracic Disease. 2015;**7**(11):E537-EE40

[8]   Thiese MS. Observational and interventional study design types; an overview. Biochemia Medica. 2014;**24**(2):199-210

[9]   Miller AB, Goff DC, BammannDr K, Wild P. Cohort Studies. In: Ahrens W, Pigeot I, editors. Handbook of Epidemiology. New York, NY: Springer; 2014. pp. 259-291

[10]  Gamble J-M. An introduction to the fundamentals of cohort and case–control studies. The Canadian Journal of Hospital Pharmacy. 2014;**67**(5):366-372

[11]  Carlson MDA, Morrison RS. Study design, precision, and validity in observational studies. Journal of Palliative Medicine. 2009;**12**(1):77-82

[12]  De Rango P. Prospective cohort studies. European Journal of Vascular and Endovascular Surgery. 2016;**51**(1):151

[13]  Costantino G, Montano N, Casazza G. When should we change our clinical practice based on the results of a clinical study? The hierarchy of evidence. Internal and Emergency Medicine. 2015;**10**(6):745-747

[14]  Burns PB, Rohrich RJ, Chung KC. The levels of evidence and their role in evidence-based medicine. Plastic and Reconstructive Surgery. 2011;**128**(1):305-310

[15]  Petrisor BA, Bhandari M. The hierarchy of evidence: Levels and grades of recommendation. Indian Journal of Orthopaedics. 2007;**41**(1):11-15

[16]  Perry-Parrish C, Dodge R. Research and statistics: Validity hierarchy for study design and study type. Pediatrics in Review. 2010;**31**(1):27-29

[17]  Murad MH, Asi N, Alsawas M, Alahdab F. New evidence pyramid. Evidence-Based Medicine. 2016

[18]  Euser AM, Zoccali C, Jager KJ, Dekker FW. Cohort studies: Prospective versus retrospective. Nephron Clinical practice. 2009;**113**(3):c214-c217

[19]  Noordzij M, Dekker FW, Zoccali C, Jager KJ. Study designs in clinical research. Nephron Clinical Practice. 2009;**113**(3):c218-cc21

[20]  Levin KA. Study design IV: Cohort studies. Evidence-Based Dentistry. 2006;**7**:51

[21]  Munnangi S, Boktor SW. Epidemiology, Study Design. Treasure Island (FL): StatPearls Publishing LLC; 2017

[22]  Setia MS. Methodology Series Module 1: Cohort Studies. Indian Journal of Dermatology. 2016;**61**(1):21-25

[23]  Merrill RM. Introduction to Epidemiology. 6th ed. Burlington, MA: Jones & Bartlett Learning; 2012

[24]  Song JW, Chung KC. Observational studies: cohort and case-control studies. Plastic and Reconstructive Surgery. 2010;**126**(6):2234-2242

[25] Grimes DA, Schulz KF. Bias and causal associations in observational research. Lancet. 2002;**359**(9302):248-252

[26] Jekel JF. Epidemiology, Biostatistics, and preventive medicine. 3rd ed. Philadelphia: Saunders/Elsevier, c2007; 2007

[27] Hulley SB, Cummings SR, Browner WS, Grady DG, Newman TB. Designing Clinical Research. Wolters Kluwer/Lippincott Williams & Wilkins; 2013

[28] Sedgwick P. Retrospective cohort studies: advantages and disadvantages. BMJ: British Medical Journal. 2014;**348**

[29] Kip KE, Cohen F, Cole SR, Wilhelmus KR, Patrick DL, Blair RC, et al. Recall bias in a prospective cohort study of acute time-varying exposures: example from the herpetic eye disease study. Journal of Clinical Epidemiology. 2001;**54**(5):482-487

[30] White E, Hunt JR, Casso D. Exposure measurement in cohort studies: the challenges of prospective data collection. Epidemiologic Reviews. 1998;**20**(1):43-56

[31] Hess DR. Retrospective studies and chart reviews. Respiratory Care. 2004;**49**(10):1171

[32] Sedgwick P. Prospective cohort studies: Advantages and disadvantages. BMJ: British Medical Journal. 2013;**347**

[33] Voormolen N, Noordzij M, Grootendorst DC, Beetz I, Sijpkens YW, van Manen JG, et al. High plasma phosphate as a risk factor for decline in renal function and mortality in pre-dialysis patients. Nephrology, dialysis, transplantation : official publication of the European Dialysis and Transplant Association - European Renal Association 2007;**22**(10):2909-2916

[34] Friberg L, Benson L, Rosenqvist M, Lip GYH. Assessment of female sex as a risk factor in atrial fibrillation in Sweden: Nationwide retrospective cohort study. BMJ: British Medical Journal. 2012;**344**

[35] Lindenauer PK, Rothberg MB, Pekow PS, Kenwood C, Benjamin EM, Auerbach AD. Outcomes of care by hospitalists, general internists, and family physicians. The New England Journal of Medicine. 2007;**357**(25):2589-2600

[36] Goodwin KA, Goodwin CJ. Research in Psychology: Methods and Design. 8th ed. Hoboken, NJ: Wiley; 2017

[37] Trochim W, Donnelly JP. The Research Methods Knowledge Base. 3rd ed. Boston, MA: Cengage Learning; 2006

[38] Sedgwick P. Bias in observational study designs: Prospective cohort studies. BMJ: British Medical Journal. 2014;**349**

[39] Hammer GP, du Prel J-B, Blettner M. Avoiding bias in observational studies: Part 8 in a series of articles on evaluation of scientific publications. Deutsches Ärzteblatt International. 2009;**106**(41):664-668

[40] Boyko EJ. Observational research--Opportunities and limitations. Journal of Diabetes and its Complications. 2013;**27**(6):642-648

[41] Sessler DI, Imrey PB. Clinical research methodology 2: Observational clinical research. Anesthesia & Analgesia. 2015;**121**(4):1043-1051

[42] Dettori JR. Loss to follow-up. Evidence-Based Spine-Care Journal. 2011;**2**(1):7-10

[43] Schoenbach V, Rosamond W. Understanding the Fundamentals of Epidemiology: An Evolving Text. University of North Carolina at Chapel Hill; 2000

[44] von Elm E, Altman DG, Egger M, Pocock SJ, Gøtzsche PC, Vandenbroucke JP. The Strengthening the Reporting of Observational Studies in Epidemiology (STROBE) statement: Guidelines for reporting observational studies. Preventive Medicine. 2007; **45**(4):247-251

[45] Vandenbroucke JP, von Elm E, Altman DG, Gøtzsche PC, Mulrow CD, Pocock SJ, et al. Strengthening the Reporting of Observational Studies in Epidemiology (STROBE): Explanation and elaboration. PLoS Medicine. 2007;**4**(10):e297

[46] Vandenbroucke JP, Elm E, Altman DG, et al. Strengthening the reporting of observational studies in epidemiology (strobe): Explanation and elaboration. Annals of Internal Medicine. 2007;**147**(8):W-163-WW-94

[47] Vandenbroucke JP, von Elm E, Altman DG, Gøtzsche PC, Mulrow CD, Pocock SJ, et al. Strengthening the Reporting of Observational Studies in Epidemiology (STROBE): Explanation and elaboration. Epidemiology 2007;**18**(6):805-835

[48] Bookwala A, Hussain N, Bhandari M. The three-minute appraisal of a prospective cohort study. Indian Journal of Orthopaedics. 2011;**45**(4):291-293

[49] Tooth L, Ware R, Bain C, Purdie DM, Dobson A. Quality of reporting of observational longitudinal research. American Journal of Epidemiology. 2005;**161**(3):280-288

[50] FHS. History of the Framingham Heart Study 2017. Available from: https://www.framinghamheartstudy.org/about-fhs/history.php

[51] Long MT, Fox CS. The Framingham Heart Study--67 years of discovery in metabolic disease. Nature Reviews Endocrinology. 2016;**12**(3):177-183

[52] Oppenheimer GM. Framingham Heart Study: the first 20 years. Progress in Cardiovascular Diseases. 2010;**53**(1):55-61

[53] Dawber TR, Meadors GF, Moore FE. Epidemiological approaches to heart disease: The Framingham Study. American Journal of Public Health and the Nations Health. 1951;**41**(3):279-286

[54] Tsao CW, Vasan RS. Cohort Profile: The Framingham Heart Study (FHS): overview of milestones in cardiovascular epidemiology. International Journal of Epidemiology. 2015;**44**(6):1800-1813

[55]  FHS. Framingham Heart Study Bibliography 2017. Available from: https://www.fram-inghamheartstudy.org/fhs-bibliography/index.php

[56]  Mahmood SS, Levy D, Vasan RS, Wang TJ. The Framingham Heart Study and the epidemiology of cardiovascular diseases: A historical perspective. Lancet. 2014; **383**(9921):999-1008

[57]  Hajar R. Framingham contribution to cardiovascular disease. Heart Views : The Official Journal of the Gulf Heart Association. 2016;**17**(2):78-81

[58]  Wilson PW, D'Agostino RB, Levy D, Belanger AM, Silbershatz H, Kannel WB. Prediction of coronary heart disease using risk factor categories. Circulation. 1998;**97**(18):1837-1847

[59]  FHS. Research Milestones 2017. Available from: https://www.framinghamheartstudy.org/about-fhs/research-milestones.php

[60]  FHS. Epidemiological Background and Design: The Framingham Study 2017. Available from: https://www.framinghamheartstudy.org/about-fhs/background.php

[61]  NHS. History 2016. Available from: http://www.nurseshealthstudy.org/about-nhs/history

[62]  NHS. About NHS 2016. Available from: http://www.nurseshealthstudy.org/about-nhs

[63]  Colditz GA, Manson JE, Hankinson SE. The Nurses' Health Study: 20-year contribution to the understanding of health among women. Journal of Women's Health. 1997;**6**(1):49-62

[64]  NHS. Key contributions to scientific knowledge 2016. Available from: http://www.nurse-shealthstudy.org/about-nhs/key-contributions-scientific-knowledge

[65]  Giovannucci E, Egan KM, Hunter DJ, Stampfer MJ, Colditz GA, Willett WC, et al. Aspirin and the risk of colorectal cancer in women. The New England Journal of Medicine. 1995;**333**(10):609-614

[66]  Baer HJ, Glynn RJ, Hu FB, Hankinson SE, Willett WC, Colditz GA, et al. Risk factors for mortality in the nurses' health study: A competing risks analysis. American Journal of Epidemiology. 2011;**173**(3):319-329

[67]  Bernstein AM, Pan A, Rexrode KM, Stampfer M, Hu FB, Mozaffarian D, et al. Dietary protein sources and the risk of stroke in men and women. Stroke. 2012;**43**(3):637-644

[68]  Chiuve SE, Fung TT, Rexrode KM, Spiegelman D, Manson JE, Stampfer MJ, et al. Adherence to a low-risk, healthy lifestyle and risk of sudden cardiac death among women. JAMA. 2011;**306**(1):62-69

[69]  Liu S, Willett WC, Stampfer MJ, Hu FB, Franz M, Sampson L, et al. A prospective study of dietary glycemic load, carbohydrate intake, and risk of coronary heart disease in US women. The American Journal of Clinical Nutrition. 2000;**71**(6):1455-1461

[70]  Hu FB, Manson JE, Stampfer MJ, Colditz G, Liu S, Solomon CG, et al. Diet, lifestyle, and the risk of type 2 diabetes mellitus in women. The New England Journal of Medicine. 2001;**345**(11):790-797

[71] Hu FB, Bronner L, Willett WC, Stampfer MJ, Rexrode KM, Albert CM, et al. Fish and omega-3 fatty acid intake and risk of coronary heart disease in women. JAMA. 2002;**287**(14):1815-1821

[72] Ayas NT, White DP, Manson JE, Stampfer MJ, Speizer FE, Malhotra A, et al. A prospective study of sleep duration and coronary heart disease in women. Archives of Internal Medicine. 2003;**163**(2):205-209

[73] Curhan GC, Willett WC, Knight EL, Stampfer MJ. Dietary factors and the risk of incident kidney stones in younger women: Nurses' Health Study II. Archives of Internal Medicine. 2004;**164**(8):885-891

[74] Holmes MD, Chen WY, Feskanich D, Kroenke CH, Colditz GA. Physical activity and survival after breast cancer diagnosis. JAMA. 2005;**293**(20):2479-2486

[75] Eliassen AH, Missmer SA, Tworoger SS, Spiegelman D, Barbieri RL, Dowsett M, et al. Endogenous steroid hormone concentrations and risk of breast cancer among premenopausal women. Journal of the National Cancer Institute. 2006;**98**(19):1406-1415

[76] Hunter DJ, Kraft P, Jacobs KB, Cox DG, Yeager M, Hankinson SE, et al. A genome-wide association study identifies alleles in FGFR2 associated with risk of sporadic postmenopausal breast cancer. Nature Genetics. 2007;**39**(7):870-874

[77] Song H, Ramus SJ, Tyrer J, Bolton KL, Gentry-Maharaj A, Wozniak E, et al. A genome-wide association study identifies a new ovarian cancer susceptibility locus on 9p22.2. Nature Genetics. 2009;**41**(9):996-1000

[78] Beral V, Doll R, Hermon C, Peto R, Reeves G. Ovarian cancer and oral contraceptives: collaborative reanalysis of data from 45 epidemiological studies including 23, 257 women with ovarian cancer and 87, 303 controls. Lancet. 2008;**371**(9609):303-314

[79] Sarwar N, Gao P, Seshasai SR, Gobin R, Kaptoge S, Di Angelantonio E, et al. Diabetes mellitus, fasting blood glucose concentration, and risk of vascular disease: A collaborative meta-analysis of 102 prospective studies. Lancet. 2010;**375**(9733):2215-2222

[80] Colditz GA, Philpott SE, Hankinson SE. The impact of the Nurses' Health Study on population health: Prevention, translation, and control. American Journal of Public Health. 2016;**106**(9):1540-1545

[81] Bristol Uo. Caerphilly Prospective Study: About 2017. Available from: https://www.bristol.ac.uk/population-health-sciences/projects/caerphilly/about/

[82] Elwood P, Galante J, Pickering J, Palmer S, Bayer A, Ben-Shlomo Y, et al. Healthy lifestyles reduce the incidence of chronic diseases and dementia: Evidence from the Caerphilly Cohort Study. PLoS One. 2013;**8**(12):e81877

[83] Mertens E, Markey O, Geleijnse JM, Lovegrove JA, Givens DI. Adherence to a healthy diet in relation to cardiovascular incidence and risk markers: evidence from the Caerphilly Prospective Study. European Journal of Nutrition. 2017

[84]  Bolton CE, Cockcroft JR, Sabit R, Munnery M, McEniery CM, Wilkinson IB, et al. Lung function in mid-life compared with later life is a stronger predictor of arterial stiffness in men: the Caerphilly Prospective Study. International Journal of Epidemiology. 2009;**38**(3):867-876

[85]  Patterson CC, Smith AE, Yarnell JW, Rumley A, Ben-Shlomo Y, Lowe GD. The associations of interleukin-6 (IL-6) and downstream inflammatory markers with risk of cardiovascular disease: The Caerphilly Study. Atherosclerosis. 2010;**209**(2):551-557

[86]  Gallacher J, Bayer A, Lowe G, Fish M, Pickering J, Pedro S, et al. Is sticky blood bad for the brain?: Hemostatic and inflammatory systems and dementia in the Caerphilly Prospective Study. Arteriosclerosis, Thrombosis, and Vascular Biology. 2010;**30**(3):599-604

[87]  Sarkar C, Gallacher J, Webster C. Built environment configuration and change in body mass index: The Caerphilly Prospective Study (CaPS). Health & Place. 2013;**19**:33-44

[88]  McEniery CM, Spratt M, Munnery M, Yarnell J, Lowe GD, Rumley A, et al. An analysis of prospective risk factors for aortic stiffness in men: 20-year follow-up from the Caerphilly prospective study. Hypertension (Dallas, Tex: 1979). 2010;**56**(1):36-43

[89]  Livingstone KM, Lovegrove JA, Cockcroft JR, Elwood PC, Pickering JE, Givens DI. Does dairy food intake predict arterial stiffness and blood pressure in men?: Evidence from the Caerphilly Prospective Study. Hypertension (Dallas, Tex: 1979). 2013;**61**(1):42-47

[90]  Eicher JD, Xue L, Ben-Shlomo Y, Beswick AD, Johnson AD. Replication and hematological characterization of human platelet reactivity genetic associations in men from the Caerphilly Prospective Study (CaPS). Journal of Thrombosis and Thrombolysis. 2016;**41**(2):343-350

[91]  Gallacher JE, Yarnell JW, Sweetnam PM, Elwood PC, Stansfeld SA. Anger and incident heart disease in the caerphilly study. Psychosomatic Medicine. 1999;**61**(4):446-453

# Chapter 3

# Limitations and Biases in Cohort Studies

Muriel Ramirez-Santana

Additional information is available at the end of the chapter

http://dx.doi.org/10.5772/intechopen.74324

### Abstract

Good practice in research involves considering diverse sources of biases when designing a study for later validation of results. If they are recognized beforehand, it is possible to minimize or avoid them. Selection biases may originate at the time of enrolling the subjects of study, making it necessary to clearly state the selection criteria of the exposed and nonexposed individuals. If people get lost from the original sample, bias may be introduced by the consequences of reducing the sample. Biases of information could originate in loss of evidence at the moment of recording the data. The definition of follow-up protocols may also help to keep registers of all variables, so information will not be missed from the individuals under study or from the observers who conduct the follow-up. It is necessary to apply the same protocols and instruments for measuring and evaluating the health outcomes in exposed and nonexposed individuals in order to avoid biases of missclassification. Confusion biases can be avoided at the time of designing the study, with the inclusion of confounding variables from the onset. Matching by age and gender is strongly recommended, and finally, adjustment techniques are used at the time of the data analysis.

**Keywords:** systematic error, selection bias, information bias, confusion, interaction, cohort studies

## 1. Introduction

The external validity of the results of an analytical study (including cohort studies) is determined by the possibility that the results can be extrapolated to larger populations, making the representativeness and randomness of the sample(s) important. However, there is controversy about the real need of representativeness when other situations are more relevant in the study, for example, some practical reasons, restrictions in the selection criteria or focus in certain population groups [1].

Internal validity, however, is determined by a series of factors that can lead to systematic errors or biases [2]. Bias can originate both in the design stage of the study, such as sample selection, data collection or analysis, but can be minimized with good planning of the study protocol or using statistical analysis techniques in this phase of the study [3]. The sample size will determine the validity in terms of the statistical power necessary to reject or approve the working hypothesis. An adequate sample size will make it easier to avoid random errors in the results of the study.

Although cohort studies have a lower risk of presenting biases than other types of epidemiological studies (ecological, cross-sectional or prevalence studies, cases and controls), they are not free of them. This chapter highlights the types of biases, their origin, their effects on the validity of the study and ways to avoid or minimize them. The chapter also gives examples that allow better understanding of the concepts as well as practical advice when carrying out a cohort study.

### 1.1. Feasibility considerations

Study protocols should always adhere to the evaluation of duly accredited Scientific Ethics Committees. Ethical principles indicate that all participants must adhere to informed consent before beginning to participate in the study, being able to understand all the implications of participating and to decline his/her participation at any moment. Authorizations of the managers in charge of the administration of any institution (healthcare centers, schools, municipalities, hospitals or others) are usually required to access the registered data or to collect the health information of the users. In studies of occupational health, authorization of the workplaces is required to perform the evaluations of jobs and workers exposed to occupational hazards. In studies about infants or children, framed in the educational sector, the assent of the minors is required, in addition to informed consent of the parents/guardians/proxies, and authorization of the executives of participating educational facilities. Collaboration agreements, purchase of laboratory services, transport, locations, surveyors, data analysis, computer support and other technical and logistical requirements that involve carrying out a follow-up study of people, usually for several years, must also be managed. When a large research team is involved, protocols must be in place for recruitment, evaluations, transporting and storage of samples and materials, laboratory procedures, recording data, backing up information and so on.

## 2. Bias in cohort studies

Certainly, among analytical epidemiological research, cohort studies are less prone to have bias than the case-control ones, specifically regarding memory bias. But as any other epidemiological study, several biases could be present in cohort studies. In this sense, researchers must be aware of those biases in advance and take them into account at the moment of selecting participants, designing the study (collection tools/instruments), when registering the data during field work (data base design) and, later on, at the moment of analyzing and interpreting the data (statistical analysis).

We understand bias as systematic errors that can lead to mistaken results or interpretation regarding the association under study, when the purpose of a study is assessing the association of certain factors toward supporting the causality of a health event or outcome [4].

There are several ways of classification of biases. For academic proposes, we will use the following classification [2, 4]:

Selection bias: originated from the way the participants of the study are selected or followed and can affect the apparent association between the exposure and outcome.

Information biases: could originate in the observed individuals, in the observers or in the instruments used to assess the outcomes.

Confusion bias: their origin is in the relationship that other variables that are not the exposition are related to the outcome, and can modulate the effect(s) of the exposition, contributing to a spurious association.

We will now review each kind of bias in detail and with some examples.

## 2.1. Selection bias

In cohort studies, the researcher must select exposed and nonexposed individuals. In the first place, it should be understood that both groups are representative of the general population from where they are taken, in order to facilitate the external validity of the study (basic condition to generalize the results in order to support causality). This condition, however, would not necessarily affect the internal validity. In other words, the internal validity is due to systematic errors sourced in stubborn participation of individuals.

The appropriated assessment of the exposure is the first crucial step. Auto-selection is one of the circumstances that could lead to inaccurate selection. As an example, a study conducted among pregnant women in Norway intended to evaluate auto-selection bias by comparing two cohorts; one group was taken from the Medical Birth Registry (2000–2006) as a population-based cohort, and the second group was from women who agreed to participate in the Norwegian Mother and Child Cohort Study. The results suggested that the prevalence estimates of exposures and the outcomes were biased due to self-selection in the Norwegian Mother and Child Cohort Study. Nevertheless, the estimates of exposure-outcome associations were not biased [5]. But in other cases, the associations could also be flawed.

Another example for selection bias might occur when the compared cohorts are part of a population who receive public health interventions, so the exposure can be misled by this influence. That is the example given by researchers who studied the association of bad water quality (measured by *E. coli* burden) and development of diarrhea in Bangladesh. Interventions to purify water (use of chlorine) may interfere by reducing the pathogens and misclassify the exposure [6].

Selection criteria must be clearly defined from the beginning of the study in a way that ensures that biases are avoided. For example, a research was conducted with the objective of assessing the association between exposure to pesticides and neurocognitive impairment, including fine motor coordination [7]. The researchers used Purdue Pegboard and MOART reaction time tests to measure the outcome. If any right- or left-handed people were selected, bias may be introduced when evaluating the outcomes due to the way that the tests are performed. Both tests have separated evaluation of left and right hands, giving certain scoring to the performance. Then, one important inclusion criterion to consider was right-handed people only; so the responses were standardized under the same criteria, and bias was eluded.

Another example of selection bias can happen in large multicenter cohort studies evaluating the association between diet and cancer. In this case, systematic errors may originate in the measurement of the exposure by dietary questionnaires that are not easy to standardize for all locations. Researchers suggest to use the calibration approach for such cases [8].

Another type of selection bias is known as the nonresponders or no-participation bias, which are less frequent in prospective cohort studies due to the need for strict following-up of the participants, strengthening the evaluations during the follow-up visits, encouraging participants and evaluators (observers) to always respond and/or register the records properly. Nevertheless, missing data could be present in retrospective cohort studies, where previously registered data are used. This will be explained in detail later, related to the information biases (Section 2.2).

In prospective cohort studies, loss of follow-up may occur, giving rise to selection bias. Loss of follow-up bias is caused by the loss of individuals from one or more exposure groups. Because cohort studies take normally several months or years of following the participants, it is expected that life situations will vary from time to time, causing some of the participants to get lost during the development of the study. Individuals can be lost homogeneously in the groups to be compared, causing bias of poor global miss-classification, which generally leads the estimate toward the null value [9]. Or individuals from a single group can be lost, causing bias of poor differential miss-classification. In the first case, the estimated risk would not be severely affected, because the incidence rates would keep similar in both groups, but the power of the results may be lost. In the latter case, the results to be obtained may be underestimating or overestimating the association. For example, if the people who are exposed and develop the outcome (disease) are lost, the incidence rate may be lower among the exposed individuals and the relative risk (RR) would be underestimated. On the other hand, if people who are not exposed and do not get the disease after time of follow-up get lost, then the incidence rate among the nonexposed will be higher and the RR would be overestimated.

Here is a hypothetic example showing the four possibilities of losing individuals:

**Original data**:

Size of the exposed cohort = 1000.

Size of the nonexposed cohort = 1000.

Number of individuals with the outcome among the exposed = 100.

Number of individuals with the outcome among the nonexposed = 10.

**Correct results:**

Incidence rate in exposed = 100/1000 = 0.1.

Incidence rate in nonexposed = 10/1000 = 0.01.

Relative risk = 10.

**Loss of 50 individuals during follow-up with the disease among the exposed:**

Incidence rate in exposed = 50/1000 = 0.05.

Incidence rate in nonexposed = 10/1000 = 0.01.

Relative risk = 5.

**Loss of five individuals during follow-up with the disease among the nonexposed:**

Incidence rate in exposed = 100/1000 = 0.1.

Incidence rate in nonexposed = 5/1000 = 0.005.

Relative risk = 20.

**Loss of 100 individuals during follow-up without the disease among the exposed:**

Incidence rate in exposed = 100/800 = 0.125.

Incidence rate in nonexposed = 10/1000 = 0.01.

Relative risk = 12.5.

**Loss of 200 individuals during follow-up without the disease among the nonexposed:**

Incidence rate in exposed = 100/1000 = 0.1.

Incidence rate in nonexposed = 10/800 = 0.0125.

Relative risk = 8.

As you can see, the estimated association variation is given by the number of people who completed the follow-up schedule. The general recommendation is that 60–80% of the individuals complete the timeframe defined originally, but a study that simulated a cohort of 500 observations with 1000 replications in computer found utterly biased estimates of the risks with low ranks of loss to follow-up [10]. On the other hand, as was already said, the results of the diminution in the number of subjects can also affect the statistical power of the results. Then, in the design of the study, at least 10% sample loss must be considered, so this proportion must be added to the minimum calculated sample size for the study. During the field work phase, measures need to be taken in advance in order to avoid losing individuals. To ensure the permanence of the individuals during the follow-up time, it is suggested to include incentives for the participants. These incentives do not necessarily have to be monetary, and a food and transportation voucher can be offered for those who attend scheduled evaluations.

In addition, it may happen that nonexposed individuals enter into the exposed group or vice versa. An example of this could occur when studying the association of tobacco consumption and a certain outcome. Then, during the study, people who smoke can leave the consumption and/or people who do not smoke can start smoking. In those cases, it is suggested to use the *incidence density* indicator instead of the cumulative incidence. The incidence density is interpreted as exposure measured in units of *person-time*, for example, person-weeks or person-days. Person-time is the sum of the time periods of observation of each person who has been observed for all or part of the entire time period [4].

The incidence density is calculated as follows:

$$\frac{\text{Number of new cases of a disease occurring in a population during a specified period of time}}{\text{Total person} - \text{time (the sum of the time periods of observation of each person who was observed for all or part of the entire time period)}} \times 1.000. \quad (1)$$

It is important to mention that the person-time unit is not in all occasions equivalent to the person-time of all individuals. For example, one person-year could represent one person being followed for 1 year or two people being followed for 6 months. But in any case, this is a way of measuring incidence that is very useful in cohort studies because it avoids the issue of subjects shifting form one exposure group to the other.

Finally, we have the selective survival bias. This bias is known in occupational health as the *healthy worker effect* and occurs when workers who have the health effect (disease or outcome) abandon the work, so a greater proportion of healthy exposed workers finally lead to underestimation of the health effect or outcome. This situation may happen when the exposed individuals have the condition already for certain time (prevalent cohort), so the probability to express the outcome is greater than individuals who were recently exposed (incident cohort). That effect is known as *left truncation bias* or *time related (immortal time bias, time lag bias)* [11, 12]. This influence has been described in several studies: occupational settings, development of AIDS among HIV patients, cancer survival, obstetric research, use of acetylsalicylic acid and myocardial infarction [13–15]. The last is a good example, showing how the use of a cohort recently diagnosed with myocardial infarction has differences in baseline characteristics and prognosis compared to the group that has had the disease for some time (prevalent cohort), even though they were taken from the same population. Then, the researcher suggested studying incident cohorts when estimating survival of a defined outcome [14]. Another example of occupational health has been published utilizing simulation with the Monte Carlo technique. Results showed that prevalent jobs contribute to descendant bias in an occupational cohort. This arises because individuals who are less susceptible to the exposure's effect continue to be exposed, thus undervaluing the association [13].

## 2.2. Information biases

Loss during follow-up may cause information bias that was already explained in detail in Section 2.1 [10].

Usually in prospective cohorts, information bias is easy to elude, because measures may be taken during the design by including all variables in the registration forms (instruments), in order to not miss variables of interest. On the other hand, in retrospective cohorts, already existing records may be used. In that case, there could be missing data due to poor registration quality or due to variables that were not considered to be registered in advance. In both cases, the origin of missing information can lead to information bias. To minimize this effect on large population-based cohorts, it is possible to exclude individuals who have missing data from the analyses. But, this is a decision that researchers can take when the size of the remaining cohort still allows for sufficient statistical power to validate the results. That was the case presented in a large study conducted among the Danish population assessing the association between lifestyle and colorectal cancer [16]. From a total of 160,725 potential participants, several hundreds were not included due to nonresponse, cancer diagnosis and missing data (N = 997). Finally, a cohort of over 55,000 people was included in the investigation.

One important source of bias in cohort studies can occur when diagnosing the health event or outcome. It is necessary to apply the same protocol for measuring or evaluating the health outcomes in exposed and nonexposed individuals in order to avoid the biases of misclassification [9]. Similarly to what happen in the previously explained bias caused by loss of follow-up, the final effect of misclassification will depend on whether the inaccuracy in the evaluated outcome influences both exposure groups (global misclassification bias) or only affects one of them (differential misclassification bias).

Let us have a look at a hypothetical example in a study that evaluates the risk of having myocardial infarction due to exposure to a high-fat diet. **Table 1** shows the correct classification.

If the evaluation of the exposure is misled in both groups due to the mistakes in the daily food register, this results in a non-differential misclassification. Imagining that 20% of the exposed people go to the nonexposed group and 20% of nonexposed goes to the exposed group, we could have the following situation (**Table 2**).

In that case, the relative risk is diminished due to a higher incidence among the nonexposed group.

Now, suppose that the evaluators applied two diagnostic tests to the exposed that resulted in an increased diagnosis of myocardial infarction among the exposed group. This will result in a differential misclassification due to the mistaken diagnosis in the outcomes (**Table 3**).

| High-fat diet | Myocardial infarction | |
| --- | --- | --- |
| | Disease | No disease |
| Exposed | 250 | 450 |
| Nonexposed | 100 | 900 |

RR = (250/700)/(100/1000) = 0.357/0.1 = 3.57.

**Table 1.** High-fat diet and acute myocardial infarction, *correct classification.*

| High-fat diet | Myocardial infarction | |
| --- | --- | --- |
| | Disease | No disease |
| Exposed | 290 | 410 |
| Nonexposed | 260 | 740 |
| RR = (290/700)/(260/1000) = 0.414/0.26 = 1.59. | | |

**Table 2.** High-fat diet and acute myocardial infarction, non-differential misclassification.

| High-fat diet | Myocardial infarction | |
| --- | --- | --- |
| | Disease | No disease |
| Exposed | 295 | 405 |
| Nonexposed | 100 | 900 |
| RR = (295/700)/(100/1000) = 0.421/0.1 = 4.21. | | |

**Table 3.** High-fat diet and acute myocardial infarction, differential misclassification.

In this last case, when 10% of the exposed people without myocardial infarction moved to the disease group, the result is a higher relative risk due to a higher incidence among the exposed group.

A good example of this kind of misclassification bias could be given regarding the use of mortality records, which are frequently used in epidemiological studies. The registered codes of the diagnoses may be mistaken and lead to misclassification of the outcomes. That was studied recently by Deckert, who reported the results of a simulation study based on real data of cardiovascular disease mortality [17]. He reported that non-differential bias can to lead to a null hypothesis, whereas differential misclassification leads the observed Standardized Mortality Ratios to be incorrect, in either direction or magnitude. Differences were from 10 to 30%, depending on the sensitivity and specificity characteristics of the diagnosis of cardiovascular disease [17]. Statistic techniques like quantitative bias analysis (QBA) or bootstrapping disease status imputation could be used to correct misclassification bias due to correct diagnostic codes [18]. Although statistical adjustments are possible to do in cases where standard information is available, these techniques are not always enough to overcome the bias. An example is reported by Candice Johnson et al., related to the misclassification of self-reported obesity and diabetes, adjusted by the National Health and Nutrition Examination Survey [19].

Regarding the accuracy in gathering information during the follow-up visits, one could have the temptation to assess more strictly the exposed individuals than the nonexposed or to evaluate the exposed persons more frequently than the nonexposed. The advice is to apply the same protocol and instruments to both groups of people, and in that way, bias introduced by the observer or the instruments is avoided. We understand as instruments the questionnaires, weighting scale, sphygmomanometer, altimeter, laboratory tests/techniques and others. Additionally, if the person(s) who observe and diagnose the outcome are aware of the exposure status, a preconception may lead to overdiagnose the exposed people and/or underdiagnose the nonexposed people. Alike in randomized trials, the best way to avoid this bias is blinding the observers.

There is also a possibility that bias may originate from the observed individuals. It can happen that people, who know they are under observation, change their behavior. This has been called the Hawthorne effect and is due to the effects that the research can produce in the participants (observers and/or studied individuals). This was first described in a factory near Chicago between 1924 and 1936, in which a group of workers who knew they were under strict supervision significantly improved their productivity, compared to workers who were not aware of being observed [20]. There is still some controversy about the real predisposition effect of the participant's observation and the amount of bias that could cause. Some studies have found such an effect, but others have not [20, 21]. For example, a study conducted in Tanzania regarding malaria treatment did find a modest suggestion that the health professionals maintained better practice during the study [22].

Finally, all types of epidemiological studies may be affected by partiality in the phase of the analysis. The way to avoid this analytical bias is by *masking or blinding* the statistician. That means the statistician, or the person performing the analysis, does not know the exposure condition at the time of the analysis.

## 2.3. Confusion bias and interaction

We understand a confounder as a variable that is associated with the exposure as well as to the health event or outcome, but not being necessarily a cause of the event. For example, an inaccurate causal inference can be made between drinking coffee and pancreatic cancer, when drinking coffee has been associated with a smoking habit [4]. This is known as *spurious association*.

The most common confusion variables to be considered during the design of any epidemiological study are gender and age. As cohort studies are observational, people are not randomly assigned to the exposure and nonexposure group; it is not always possible to match both groups by certain variables such as sex, age, or other confounders. Depending on the exposure or events being studied, other variables could work as confounders; therefore, before designing any study, it is important for researchers to read previous studies and develop the design with all evidence that highlight confounders.

Several examples can be given in this matter: (1) In the aforementioned study about acetylsalicylic acid exposure and major bleeding, confounders considered were age, sex, previous hospitalization for alcoholism, non-bleeding ulcer disease, other non-bleeding conditions, and comorbidities [15]; then the researchers could adjust the risk ratios according to those variables. (2) In the study relating endometriosis and infertility, the considered confounders were menstrual cycle pattern, hirsutism, participant's birthweight, race, household income, husband's education, BMI at age 18 years, alcohol consumption, oral contraception use, any analgesic use, health screening behavior, personal history of cardiovascular disease, and personal history of diabetes [23]. In that case, researchers could evaluate if any of those variables truly acted as confounders or not. (3) In a study relating air pollution and mortality risks, past exposure to pollution and habit of tobacco consumption were not considered; because they may act as confounders for the results of the association and causal inference could be misled [24]. For a better understanding, please refer to **Figure 1**.

There are some cases in which the dose of exposure may introduce confusion. Such is the case of age, smoking, or drinking alcohol. Age involves the quantity of years (or months) itself, and for the analysis, it will be possible to use as a continuous variable or create ranges of age for stratification analysis. On the other hand, for consumption, it is recommended to consider registering the quantities being consumed by the individuals, so strata can be made during the analysis phase. Tobacco may be registered by number of cigarettes per day. The case of alcohol is rather difficult. The suggestion is to ask for quantity (number of glasses) and types of drinks consumed and then transform it into grams of pure alcohol consumed daily or weekly.

Confounding variables can be controlled in several ways: restriction, matching, stratification and more sophisticated multivariate techniques [2].

Restriction is a simple way of avoiding the introduction of already known confounders, by excluding people who present that factor from the beginning. The problem is that this could

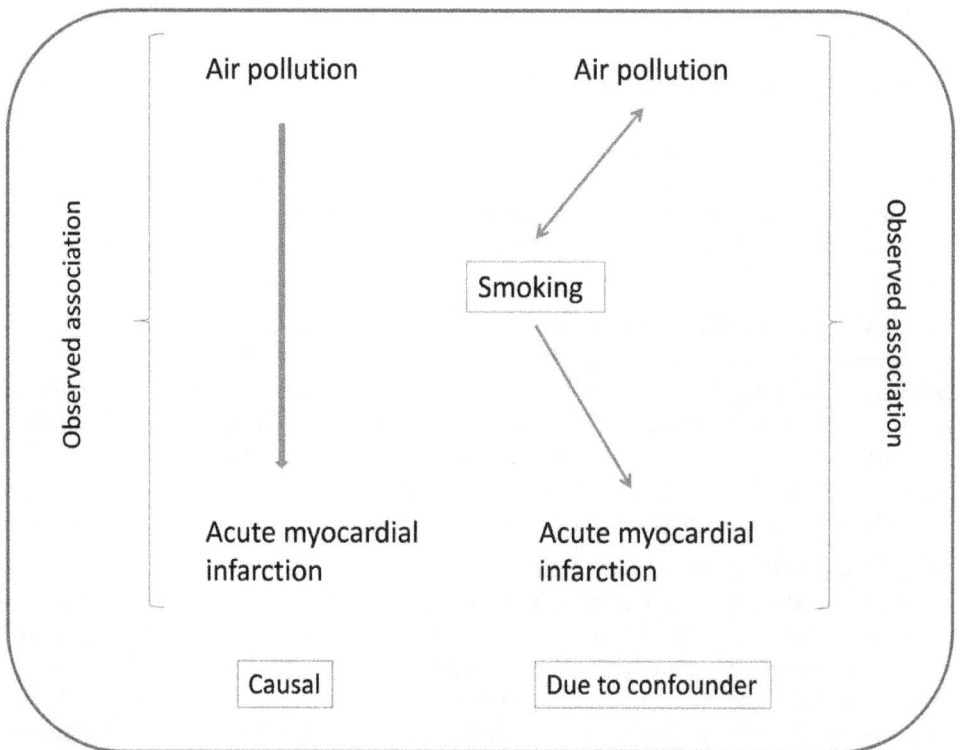

**Figure 1.** Scheme of confounding (smoking) in relation to the exposure (air pollution) and the outcome (acute myocardial infarction).

limit recruitment and the representativeness of certain population groups. So, while increasing the internal validity, this may reduce external validity [2].

As it was said before, matching is rather difficult to do in prospective studies because the first enrolment criterion is the exposure. Matching normally is used in case control studies, but researchers could emphasize that the proportion of women and men would be 50% each or that a ratio of young/old people was similar in the exposure groups.

Stratification is a simple statistic technique that could be used during analysis, but that requires forethought concerning the possible confusion variables and registering them.

The technique consists of separating the analysis of association, according to strata of the confusing factor, for example, perform separate analyses of men and women when it is suspected that gender may be a confounder. Then, when the difference between the calculated raw risk and the risk calculated by strata is over 15%, we could say that confusion is present.

Let's see an example. In a rural area, a study proposed to evaluate the relationship between indoor exposure to smoke—from the combustion of wood stoves—and the occurrence of tuberculosis (TB). The results obtained are presented in **Table 4**.

Therefore, the factor *indoor exposure to wood smoke* for food cooking turned out to be positively associated with the disease. In other words, the incidence of the disease among the exposed group was significantly more than two times greater than that among the nonexposure group.

Given that there is a suspicion that cigarette smoking could modify the effect of indoor contamination on the risk of acquiring tuberculosis, smoking habits were considered. Then, it was possible to assess if this condition acted as a confounder in the association between tuberculosis and indoor smoke exposure using stratification.

The stratification is shown below, where the smoking habit was coded as "never" or "past or present" (**Tables 5** and **6**).

As a conclusion of the stratification results, the factor *indoor exposure to smoke* was found to be positively and significantly associated with the disease, both in nonsmokers and in past or present smokers. However, in past or present smokers, the risk of suffering from tuberculosis is 44% higher than in nonsmokers (from 2.57 to 2.12), when the indoor pollution was present, confirming that smoking habit acts like a confounder in the association between indoor smoke and tuberculosis incidence.

| Indoor exposure to smoke | Tuberculosis | | |
| --- | --- | --- | --- |
| | Disease | No disease | Total |
| Exposed | 50 | 21 | 71 |
| Nonexposed | 238 | 524 | 762 |
| Total | 288 | 545 | 833 |

The RR calculation is presented as: RR = (50/71)/(238/762) = 0.704/0.312 = 2.25.

**Table 4.** Tuberculosis and indoor exposure to smoke from wood burning.

| Indoor exposure to smoke | Tuberculosis | | |
| --- | --- | --- | --- |
| | Disease | No disease | Total |
| Exposed | 33 | 17 | 50 |
| Nonexposed | 186 | 411 | 597 |

Risk ratio calculation among *never smokers*: RR = (33/50)/(186/597) = 0.66/0.311 = 2.12.

**Table 5.** TB and indoor exposure to smoke from wood burning of *never smokers*.

| Indoor exposure to smoke | Tuberculosis | | |
| --- | --- | --- | --- |
| | Disease | No disease | Total |
| Exposed | 17 | 4 | 21 |
| Nonexposed | 52 | 113 | 165 |

Risk ratio calculation among *smokers past or present*: RR = (17/21)/(52/165) = 0.81/0.315 = 2.57.

**Table 6.** TB and indoor exposure to smoke from wood burning of *past or present smokers*.

| Smoking past or present | Tuberculosis | | |
| --- | --- | --- | --- |
| | Disease | No disease | Total |
| Yes | 52 | 113 | 165 |
| No smoking | 186 | 411 | 597 |

Risk calculation of smoking among nonexposed to smoke from wood burning: RR = (52/165)/(186/597) = 0.315/0.311 = 1.01.

**Table 7.** TB and smoking habits (without indoor exposure to smoke from wood burning).

In addition to confusion, we have the concept of *interaction* that refers to the effect that two of more factors have by increasing or reducing the incidence of a disease when they are together. Then, the incidence resulting when the factors are together differs from the incidence when the factors are isolated.

Let us try to find interaction in the same example.

In order to assess interaction, it will be necessary to calculate the association between smoking and tuberculosis alone (without the indoor exposure to wood burning smoke) **Table 7**.

The result shows that the relative risk of developing TB due exclusively to the habit of smoking is almost nil. But, to know if there is interaction, we should estimate if the presence of both exposures together differs or not from the expected effects if the two exposures were simply the sum of both.

From the previous tables and calculations, we have that the incidences are the following:

- Incidence rate of TB without any smoke exposure = 31.1%

- Incidence rate of TB with smoking only = 31.5%

- Incidence rate of TB with indoor pollution only = 66%

- Incidence rate of TB with smoking and indoor pollution = 81%

In order to know whether interaction is present, we should clear the incidences from the underground risk of developing TB (baseline incidence). Then, we should start by calculating the attributable risks (ARs), as follows:

AR to smoking = (TB incidence due to smoking−baseline TB incidence) = 31.5–31.1 = 0.4.

AR to indoor pollution = (TB incidence if indoor pollution−baseline TB incidence) = 66–31.1 = 34.9.

The expected attributable risk to both factors would be the addition of the TB incidence of (smoking + indoor contamination) = 34.9 + 0.4 = 35.3%. Then, the expected incidence will be (31.1 + 35.3) = 66.4%.

But the real TB incidence with both exposure factors was 81%. The difference between 81 and 66.4 would be attributable to the interaction, which is 14.6%.

In other way, the incidence when both factors are together is higher than the addition of incidences when the factors are alone, taking into consideration that we have to clear the underground risk (incidence of TB in population free of exposures).

Effectively, we have shown that interaction is present, because the incidences of both exposures together differ from the expected effects if the two exposures were simply the sum of both. As a conclusion, the indoor pollution is a risk factor to develop TB in that setting, but this risk increases substantially more if people smoke indoors. For a better understanding, please refer to **Figure 2**.

Coming back to the control of confusion bias, adjustment techniques using statistical models require computer training and have the advantage of working with two or more possible confounding variables; opposite to stratification that permits working on one factor only. When using modeling multivariate techniques, logistic regression or proportional hazard regression might be used, but researchers must be aware of how to interpret the results properly [2].

An important comment about the confusion is that finding a confounder is not always an issue to be worried about. It could also be useful. For example, in the mentioned study about pesticide exposure in agricultural workers and cognitive impairment, gender turned out to be a confounder [7]. This resulted from the type of work performed differing between men and women. Men used to perform tasks like mixing, blending and applying pesticides; while women proned to collecting fruits, so men were directly exposed to the toxins. Then, knowing that men were more exposed and, consequently, more susceptible to the health damage, the preventive measures may be oriented by strengthening them toward men, but still keeping care on women.

Finally, confounders are not a mistake in the research, but a phenomenon that is present must be understood by the investigators in order to finally consider them when interpreting the results of the study [4].

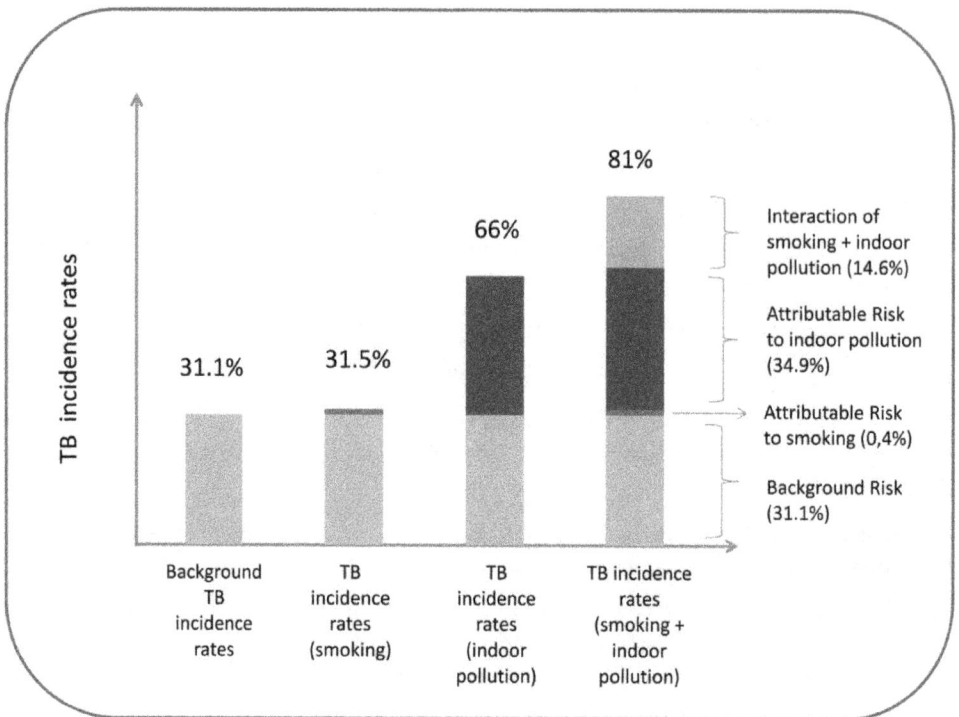

**Figure 2.** Incidence rates and attributable risk to factors related to TB incidence and their interaction.

## 3. Conclusions

As shown, biases can be present in any study, originating from multiple steps of the investigation. Their presence should not be grounds for rejection of the results due to the poor quality of the study, but careful attention is required when interpreting the results. To the extent that the researcher is able to recognize the biases, he/she can be proactive in mitigating them, either by way of improving the design or applying statistical techniques (stratification or multivariate adjustment) when analyzing the results. Therefore, when clinicians or researchers look for good quality of articles to read and use as references, they must recognize them when interpreting the results and acknowledge the limitations that the studies may have.

It should be noted that biases are more frequent among retrospective cohort, given by missing information when using existing records (information bias) or by selection bias, because individuals are selected after the outcome has occurred, so both conditions (exposure and outcome) are present at the moment of enrollment. In that case, it is easier that exposed or unexposed subjects would be related to the result of interest, causing selection bias. On the other hand, a prospective cohort design could be affected by the loss of follow-up. Both types of cohort studies may be influenced by information bias, confusion or interaction.

Interesting tools for weighting quality and predisposition to unfairness in observational studies have been gathered and reported by Sanderson et al. [25]. Those included items for selection methods, measurement of study variables, design-specific sources of bias, control of confounding variables and use of statistics.

Finally, it is considered that cohort studies are used normally as a source of information of systematic reviews and meta-analysis. In those cases, publication bias and outcome reporting bias must be taken into consideration. This is because the journals are prone to publish positive results rather than negative ones, a situation that has been shown [26].

## Conflict of interest

The author of this chapter declares no conflict of interest.

## Author details

Muriel Ramirez-Santana

Address all correspondence to: mramirezs@ucn.cl

Public Health Department, Faculty of Medicine, Universidad Catolica del Norte, Coquimbo, Chile

## References

[1] Richiardi L, Pizzi C, Pearce N. Commentary: Representativeness is usually not necessary and often should be avoided. International Journal of Epidemiology. 2017;**42**:1018-1022

[2] Grimes DA, Schulz KF. Bias and causal associations in observational research. Lancet. 2002;**359**:248-252

[3] Mantel N. Avoidance of bias in cohort studies. National Cancer Institute Monograph. May 1985;**67**:169-172

[4] Gordis L. Epidemiology. 4th ed. Philadelphia: Elsevier; 2009

[5] Roy MN, Vollset SE, Gjessing HK, Skjærven R, Melve KK, Schreuder P, Alsaker ER, Haug K, Daltveit AK, Per Magnus. Self selection bias in a large prospective pregnancy cohort in Norway. Paediatric and Perinatal Epidemiology 2009;**23**:507-608

[6] Ercumen A, Arnold BF, Naser AM, Unicomb L, Colford JM, Luby SP. Potential sources of bias in the use of Escherichia coli to measure waterborne diarrhoea risk in low-income settings. Tropical Medicine & International Health. 2017;**22**:2-11

[7] Ramírez-Santana M, Zúñiga L, Corral S, Sandoval R, Scheepers PT, Van Der Velden K, Roeleveld N, Pancetti F. Assessing biomarkers and neuropsychological outcomes in rural populations exposed to organophosphate pesticides in Chile—Study design and protocol Environmental and occupational health. BMC Public Health. 2015;15:116. DOI: 10.1186/s12889-015-1463-5

[8] Kaaks R, Plummer M, Riboli E, Estève J, Van Staveren W. Adjustment for bias due to errors in exposure assessments in multicenter cohort studies on diet and cancer: A calibration approach. The American Journal of Clinical Nutrition. 1994;59:2455-2505

[9] Copeland KT, Checkoway H, McMichael AJ, Holbrook RH. Bias due to misclassification in the estimation of relative risk. American Journal of Epidemiology. 1997;105(5):188-495. DOI: https://doi.org/10.1093/oxfordjournals.aje.a112408

[10] Kristman V, Manno M, Côte P. Loss to follow-up in cohort studies: how much is too much? European Journal of Epidemiology. 2004;19:751-760

[11] Lévesque Linda E, Hanley James A, Kezouh Abbas SS. Problem of immortal time bias in cohort studies: Example using statins for preventing progression of diabetes. British Medical Journal. 2010;340:b5087. DOI: https://doi.org/10.1136/bmj.b5087

[12] Suissa S. Lower risk of death with SGLT2 inhibitors in observational studies: Real or bias? Diabetes Care. Jan. 2018;41:6-10

[13] Applebaum KM, Malloy EJ, Eisen EA. Left truncation, susceptibility, and bias in occupational cohort studies. NIH Public Access. 2014;22:599-606

[14] Buckley BS, Simpson CR, McLernon DJ, Hannaford PC, Murphy AW. Considerable differences exist between prevalent and incident myocardial infarction cohorts derived from the same population. Journal of Clinical Epidemiology. 2010;63:1351-1357

[15] Pedersen L, Stürmer T. Conditioning on future exposure to define study cohorts can induce bias: The case of low-dose acetylsalicylic acid and risk of major bleeding. Clinical Epidemiology. 2017;9:611-626

[16] Sedgwick P. Cohort studies: Souce of bias. British Medical Journal. 2011;343:d7839. DOI: https://doi.org/10.1136/bmj.d7839

[17] Deckert A. The existence of standard-biased mortality ratios due to death certificate misclassification - A simulation study based on a true story. BMC Medical Research Methodology. 2016;16:1-9

[18] Walraven C. A comparison of methods to correct for misclassification bias from administrative database diagnostic codes. International Journal of Epidemiology. 2017;0:1-12

[19] Johnson CY, Flanders WD, Strickland MJ, Honein MA, Howards PP. Potential sensitivity of bias analysis results to incorrect assumptions of nondifferential or differential binary exposures misclassification. Epidemiology. 2014;15:902-909

[20] McCambridge J, Witton J, Elbourne DR. Systematic review of the Hawthorne effect: New concepts are needed to study research participation effects. Journal of Clinical Epidemiology. 2014;**67**:267-277

[21] Henry SG, Jerant A, Iosif A-M, Feldman MD, Cipri C, Kravitz RL. Analysis of threats to research validity introduced by audio recording clinic visits: Selection bias, Hawthorne effect, both, or neither? Diagnostic Microbiology and Infectious Disease. 2016;**28**:1304-1314

[22] Leurent B, Reyburn H, Muro F, Mbakilwa H, Schellenberg D. Monitoring patient care through health facility exit interviews: An assessment of the Hawthorne effect in a trial of adherence to malaria treatment guidelines in Tanzania. BMC Infectious Diseases. 2016; **16**(59):1-9

[23] Prescott J, Farland LV, Tobias DK, Gaskins AJ, Spiegelman D, Chavarro JE, Rich-Edwards JW, Barbieri RL, Missmer SA. A prospective cohort study of endometriosis and subsequent risk of infertility. Human Reproduction. 2016;**31**:1475-1482

[24] Hansell A, Ghosh RE, Blangiardo M, Perkins C, Vienneau D, Goffe K, Briggs D, Gulliver J. Historic air pollution exposure and Long-term mortality risks in England and Wales: Prospective longitudinal cohort study. Thorax. 2016;**71**:330-338

[25] Sanderson S, Tatt ID, Higgins JPT. Tools for assessing quality and susceptibility to bias in observational studies in epidemiology : A systematic review and annotated bibliography. International Journal of Epidemiology. 2007;**36**:666-676

[26] Dwan K, Altman DG, Arnaiz JA, et al. Systematic Review of the empirical evidence of study publication bias and outcome reporting bias. PLoS One. 2008;**3**:1-30

# Chapter 4

# Cohort Studies in the Understanding of Chronic Musculoskeletal Pain

Cristhian Saavedra Santiesteban

Additional information is available at the end of the chapter

http://dx.doi.org/10.5772/intechopen.75517

### Abstract

Chronic pain is an important clinical and social problem worldwide, affecting one in every five people. It generates a large economic burden on the health system and million dollar losses in the socio-labour field, and also directly impacts the health and quality of life of people by generating different levels of disability. Nowadays, it has been shown that this clinical manifestation is influenced by biological, psychological and social components, creating a complex scenario when proposing an effective therapeutic intervention. In consideration of this reality, we present a review of the available scientific evidence regarding the contributions that cohort studies provide for understanding chronic musculoskeletal pain, with the aim of identifying risk factors, prognostic factors and rehabilitation.

**Keywords:** chronic pain, cohort studies, risk factors, prognosis, physical therapy, rehabilitation

## 1. Introduction

Chronic pain is an important clinical, social and economic problem worldwide [1]. It is a common problem that entails a series of consequences affecting the quality of life of those patients afflicted with chronic pain, along with the difficulty placed on the health system due to the various benefits provided, producing permanent economic conflicts [2].

This reality leads to the constant pilgrimage of patients through various medical specialties, physical medicine and rehabilitation services, excessive and varied consumption of drugs that together have highly unsatisfactory results, thus producing a hopeless scenario for people with chronic musculoskeletal pain [3].

Therefore, the governments of each country are concerned about finding means that provide a solution for this situation, searching and promoting different strategies for the health system [4].

This demand for assistance has proved a great challenge for the worldwide scientific community, where they must focus their efforts on finding and providing evidence for a better understanding of the nature of chronic pain and its intervening mechanisms; seeking to contribute to the development of effective health interventions, both preventive and curative.

Pain is a complex clinical manifestation, difficult to describe fully, especially when it becomes persistent and disabling. Therefore, defining the experience of each individual and reaching a full consensus on the matter is not easy. The understanding of pain has been a subject of extensive discussion, especially over the last two decades where exponential advances have been made.

The International Association for the Study of Pain (IASP) defines it as an unpleasant sensory and emotional experience associated with actual or potential tissue damage or described in terms of such damage [5].

The World Health Organization classifies the pain as acute, chronic malignant and chronic non-malignant, incorporating chronic musculoskeletal pain in the latter.

Chronic musculoskeletal pain is conceptualized in diverse ways; either as pain that lasts for more than 3 months or pain that exceeds the time of tissue recovery. It is also known as pain that lasts for more than 6 months [5].

## 1.1. Epidemiology of chronic pain

The prevalence of chronic pain is on average 20% worldwide [6], but the numbers are variable depending on different factors such as, the methodology used in each study, the region or country analyzed and the age range; it fluctuates between 2 and 50% [2]. The prevalence of chronic pain in adults is in the range 12–42% worldwide [7].

In Europe, non-oncological chronic pain in 2011 fluctuated between 10 and 30%. In 2013, an estimated 20% of adults suffered from chronic pain [2].

In the USA, the reported frequency of chronic pain in women is 34.3 and 26.7% in men, increasing with age, and with lumbar pain being the most frequent cause (8.1%, followed by osteoarthritis 3.9%). During the year 2010, the National Health Interview Survey reported that 39.4 million American adults suffered from persistent pain of which 67.2% manifested constant pain and 50.5% reported unbearable pain [7, 8].

In 2001, the Australian population presented a prevalence of 17.1% in men and 20% in women, increasing to 27% in women between 65 and 69 years, with a peak of 31% in the age range of 80–84 years [9].

A study in 2005 reported that in Spain, the prevalence of chronic pain ranged between 10.1 and 55.2%, with a higher incidence in women [10]. On the other hand, in 2002, a study estimated a prevalence of 23.4%, where 23% were rheumatological diseases (7 million people) and 50% comprised work disabilities [11, 12].

Regarding chronic pain in the elderly population, in Sweden in 2016, the prevalence was 38.5%, being more common in women and in the age range 85–94 years, with an incidence of 5.4% per year [13]. In 2013, in the United States, the prevalence in older adults ranged between 27 and 86%, and between 13.3 and 20% patients developed pain after 3 to 6 years.

In children and adolescents, the prevalence of back pain for longer than 3 months ranges from 18 to 24% [1, 7, 14].

## 1.2. The economic impact of chronic pain

Considering the high healthcare demand generated by chronic musculoskeletal pain, added to the functional limitations and disability that this entails, chronic pain involves a high economic cost and diverse social consequences.

In Australia, the impact of lumbar spine disorders on the labour force generates a loss of AU $ 4.8 billion per year. Estimating that people with chronic moderate–severe pain lose an average of 8 work days every 6 months, the government spends millions in additional payments for welfare and large losses in tax revenues, adding annually AU $ 2.9 billion in losses of internal product gross (GDP) [15].

It is estimated that older Australians who do not work due to poor health, reduce the GDP by 14.7 billion per year, with lumbar pain and arthritis responsible for half of this burden [16].

The total indirect and direct costs resulting from adolescents with chronic pain in the United Kingdom is approximately £8.000 per year [17].

In Europe, chronic pain produces a total estimated cost of 1.5 to 3.0 of the GDP [18].

In Belgium, the cost for the health system only for back pain ranges between € 83.8 and € 164.7 trillion per year, in the UK £1 trillion, and Germany €5.11 trillion [1, 6].

In 2010 in the USA, the total costs resulting from chronic pain varied between $560 and $635 billion, exceeding the annual costs produced by heart disease, cancer and diabetes [7].

Consequently, it is clear that we are facing a large clinical and socio-economic problem; the pandemic nature of chronic pain has been difficult to control by health services throughout the world.

Despite its great impact, therapeutic approaches and rehabilitation for people with chronic musculoskeletal pain is still a pending issue and remains an important challenge to the scientific field. Although scientific advances have reoriented therapeutic approaches, there is still a great need to strengthen knowledge and provide greater support to the clinical field.

There are various interventions and factors that act on pain and that deserve to be studied through analytical and observational designs to deepen our knowledge in this field.

Consequently, this chapter proposes to review the available scientific evidence from cohort studies, emphasizing their importance and contribution to understanding chronic musculo-skeletal pain, the identification of risk factors, associated prognostic factors, visualizing the development of follow-ups after rehabilitation interventions, assessing the clinical impact of the delivered evidence, and also trying to identify the components that can contribute to daily clinical practice.

Observational studies can provide more information than clinical studies in diverse compo-nents due to the multifactorial and multidimensional nature of pain.

## 2. Cohort studies of chronic musculoskeletal pain

Cohort studies allow us to identify the behaviour of different factors that can influence chronic musculoskeletal pain over the course of time, such as risk factors, protective factors and prognostic factors, as well as observe the short and long term results of a specific therapeutic intervention.

### 2.1. Risk, protector and prognostic factors in chronic pain

In this review, it can be observed that the research found mainly focus on the study of pain in high prevalence musculoskeletal disorders, such as generalized musculoskeletal pain, chronic lower back pain syndrome (LBPS), and whiplash (**Table 1**). The risk factors observed were stress, anxiety, fear of movement, fear-avoidance behaviors, catastrophic beliefs of pain, pain intensity, depressive symptoms, psychological distress, somatisation, perceived physical exer-tion, traumas, critical life events, co-morbidities, smoking and obesity.

As protective and prognostic factors, we find self-efficacy, active pain coping, resilience, self-perception of health, social support at work, quality of sleep, stress and anxiety control, level of disability related to pain, acceptance of pain, body awareness, behaviour, quality of life related to health, recovery expectations, classification by subgroups of risk, influence of a healthy lifestyle, self-perception of prognosis and high uric acid plasma concentrations.

#### 2.1.1. Generalized chronic pain (GCP)

GCP is a common symptom of musculoskeletal pain, especially in older adults. This condition often has an important impact on functional capacity, generating different disability levels.

Since the elder population is prone to developing fragility due to different factors, a longitu-dinal study performed over an average of 4.3 years of a cohort of 2736 European men recruited from cities in eight countries (Florence (Italy), Leuven (Belgium), Lodz (Poland), Malmo (Sweden), Manchester (United Kingdom), Santiago de Compostela (Spain), Szeged (Hungary) and Tartu (Estonia)), showed that people with GCP were significantly more likely to develop or increase fragility, independent of previously identified risk factors such as smoking or alcohol consumption. Therefore, a comprehensive evaluation of elderly people

| Reference | Sample | Follow-up time | Factors related to pain | Measurement | Instrument | Outcomes |
|---|---|---|---|---|---|---|
| Fredrika et al., 2016 | 2.736 | 4.3 years | Chronic pain and frailty | Frailty | Frailty index (FI) | Among men who were non-frail at baseline, those with chronic widespread pain were significantly more likely to develop frailty. |
| | | | | Depression | Beck's Depression Inventory-II (BDI-II) | |
| | | | | Quality of life | 36-Item Medical Outcomes Study Survey (SF-36) | |
| | | | | | | After adjustment for age and centre, compared with those with no pain, those with Chronic widespread pain at baseline had a 70% higher frailty index at follow-up |
| | | | | Physical activity | Physical Activity Scale for the Elderly (PASE) | |
| | | | | Physical performance | Physical Performance Test (PPT) | |
| | | | | Balance and postural stability | Tinetti's balance and postural stability index | |
| Melloh et al. [24] | 315 | 6 months | Pain prognostic occupational factors | Location of pain | Body pain drawing | Social support at work should be considered as a resource preventing the development of persistent LBP (an overall predictive value of 78%). Somatization should be considered as a risk factor for the development of persistent LBP. |
| | | | | | Model from Pfau et al. | |
| Andersen et al. [20] | 4.977 | 3 years | Perceived physical exertion during healthcare work | Perceived exertion | Borg's rate perceived exertion scale (RPE) | Female healthcare workers with light perceived physical exertion during healthcare work have a better prognosis for recovery from long-term pain in the low back and neck/shoulders |
| | | | | Musculoskeletal symptoms | Standardized Nordic Questionnaire | |
| Bohman et al. [25] | 8.994 | 4 years | Influence of the behavior of a healthy lifestyle in the prognosis of the lower back pain | Musculoskeletal symptoms | Standardized Nordic Questionnaire | The risk was reduced by 35% for women with one healthy lifestyle factor and 52% for women with all four healthy lifestyle factors |
| | | | | Healthy lifestyle behaviour | Self-report questionnaire on healthy lifestyle behaviour | |

| Reference | Sample | Follow-up time | Factors related to pain | Measurement | Instrument | Outcomes |
|---|---|---|---|---|---|---|
| Williamson et al. [26] | 599 | 12 months | Risk factors for chronic disability in patients with acute whiplash associated disorders seeking. | Neck disability | Neck Disability Index (NDI) | 30% of participants (n = 136/459) who returned their 12 month questionnaire had developed chronic disability. |
| | | | | Pain intensity | Modified Von-Korff Pain Scale | |
| | | | | Whiplash grades | The Quebec Taskforce WAD grading system | Baseline disability had the strongest association with chronic disability, also psychological and behavioral factors were important. |
| | | | | Neck of movement | | |
| | | | | Coping | Neck range of movement (ROM) | |
| | | | | Pain catastrophizing | Coping strategies questionnaire (CSQ) | The total number of risk factors present should be considered when evaluating the potential for poor outcome |
| | | | | Fear Avoidance Beliefs | The Pain Catastrophizing Scale (PCS) | |
| | | | | Coping | Fear Avoidance Beliefs Questionnaire (FABQ) | |
| | | | | | Pain coping questionnaire (PCQ) | |
| | | | | | Passive coping | |
| | | | | General Health | General Health Questionnaire (GHQ)-12 | |
| | | | | Social support | Multidimensional scale of perceived social support | |
| Andersson et al. [21] | 107 | 12 months | Increase in serum uric in chronic pain | Number of pain locations | The sum of reported areas with current pain location | A relative increase in serum uric in combination with report of a high number of pain locations turned out to be a risk factor of increased pain extension |
| | | | | Pain intensity | Visual analogue scale (VAS) | |
| | | | | Pain duration | Question on duration of current pain | Corticosteroids diminished the risk of developing an increased number of pain locations |
| | | | | Body mass index | Calculated from initial measurements of height and weight. | |

| Reference | Sample | Follow-up time | Factors related to pain | Measurement | Instrument | Outcomes |
|---|---|---|---|---|---|---|
| | | | | Alcohol consumption | An index based on frequency of intake for strong beer, red and white wine and spirits | |
| | | | | Report of stress | Multidimensional Pain Inventory (MPI) | |
| | | | | Sleeping difficulties | Multidimensional Pain Inventory (MPI) | |
| | | | | Depression | Hospital Anxiety and Depression Scale" (HADS) | |
| | | | | Use of steroid | Answer to a question on the use of steroids (oral, intramuscular or intraarticular) last month | |

**Table 1.** Risk factors in chronic pain.

with generalized pain is important to visualize the impact of musculoskeletal pain on functionality and general health wellbeing [19].

In the adult population, a prospective study with a cohort of 4977 Danish people working in the health industry sought to determine how different levels of perception of physical effort during work influence the prognosis of long-term recovery of those with pain in different regions of the body (lumbar area, neck/shoulder and knees). They concluded that a physical effort perceived as light was associated with a good long-term prognosis for pain in the lower back, but not for knee pain. A perception of moderate physical effort is associated with a poor long-term prognosis for all the regions with reported pain [20].

Another study in adult women about GCP and the increase in pain locations shows a significant correlation with the increase in uric acid plasma concentrations after a one-year follow-up, recognizing this combination as a risk factor for the expansion of inflammatory and non-inflammatory pain [21].

### 2.1.2. Chronic low back pain

Physical, psychological and behavioral components of chronic LBPS have a direct implication on the transition from acute to chronic pain. The risk factors for this transition include anxiety, depression, traumas and critical life events; meanwhile, the protective factors include resilience, coping strategies, stress management and self-efficacy.

Another study determined that depression, psychological distress, passive coping strategies and high levels of fear related to pain are predictors of a poor evolution in patients suffering from chronic LBPS [22]. They also added the knowledge of the possibility of developing chronicity at the onset of pain as another risk factor.

Self-perception of general health, considering both physical and psychosocial dimensions, plus the expectations of patient recovery, presents a strong relation for a positive evolution [23].

Additionally, assessment of the chronicity of occupational back pain discovered two predictors related to work with a predictive value of 78%. The report observed social support as a protective factor and somatisation as a risk factor for development of persistent pain. Consequently, cognitive and psychological components play a vital role in the development or control of chronic low back pain [24].

When considering the influence of a healthy lifestyle as a prognostic factor for lower back pain, a Swedish study followed a cohort of 3938 men and 5056 women over 4 years. They were classified into five levels according to the number of healthy lifestyle factors they presented (0 to 4), declaring healthy factors as: non-smoking, no alcohol risk consumption, a recommended level of recreational physical activity and recommended weekly consumption of fruits and vegetables. The study established cut-off points (healthy / unhealthy) according to the recommendations for a healthy lifestyle established by the World Health Organization (WHO). There was a decrease in the risk of developing persistent lower back pain in women who only presented occasional lower back pain; decreasing the risk by a larger proportion as more healthy factors were present. Therefore, a healthy lifestyle is an effective indication of an improved prognosis [25].

### 2.1.3. Whiplash pain

People with acute disorders associated with whiplash are exposed to a complex clinical outcome, hindering favorable evolution due to the psychological impact generated by the traumatic circumstances experienced due to the injury. In this disorder, there are a high number of risk factors, such as psychological distress, passive coping, high initial disability, intense pain and long recovery time. A longitudinal study performed in the United Kingdom identified and assessed the impact of risk factors of developing chronic disability in acute whiplash disorders. The study consisted of a cohort of 430 subjects with a history of whiplash, initially assessing risk factors on average 32 days after injury, with a follow-up 12 months later. They found that the presence of a risk factor increased the risk of developing a chronic disability by 3.5 times and the presence of four or five risk factors increased this risk 16 times. Therefore, it is evident that the disability is directly influenced by psychological factors, behavioral factors and the presence of initial disability [26].

### 2.2. Therapeutic approaches for chronic musculoskeletal pain

Cohort studies have also contributed to the development of convincing evidence useful for developing therapeutic approaches for chronic pain, indisputably supporting clinical procedures and the establishment of public health policies.

The elaboration of an effective intervention plan for the rehabilitation of chronic pain patients is a constant challenge. It is for this reason that current therapeutic strategies and procedures try to cover the different components involved in the development of this clinical situation. Based on this need, the evidence from observational studies shows different intervention measures, such as polymodal or interdisciplinary programmes, studies about the acceptance of pain, pain education programmes, the involvement of attention/distraction and self-care plans on pain, and auto-therapeutic indications that focus on self-efficacy and recovery expectations or patient-centred approaches (**Table 2**).

A therapeutic programme based on pain education showed significant improvements regarding pain intensity, disability, catastrophism, depression, anxiety and health, with few positive results on anguish and cognition [27]. Acceptance of pain, considered as the willingness to participate in various activities in the community despite the pain, has been associated as a positive mechanism regarding the intensity of the perceived pain, improvements in the

| Reference | Sample | Follow-up time | Intervention | Measurement | Instrument | Outcomes |
|---|---|---|---|---|---|---|
| Mehlsen et al. [22] | 87 | 5 months | The Chronic Pain Self-Management Programme is a lay-led patient education | Pain | Visual analog scale (VAS) | Participants showed significant improvements in pain, disability, catastrophism, depression, anxiety and health worry, and the changes remained stable during the follow-up period. |
| | | | | Pain intensity | McGill Pain Questionnaire | |
| | | | | Physical disability | Modified Roland-Morris Disability Questionnaire | |
| | | | | Pain Catastrophizing | Pain Catastrophizing Scale | A consistent pattern of stable improvements in pain, cognition of pain and distress was observed, but the scope of the changes was modest. |
| | | | | Pain-related self-efficacy | Arthritis Self efficacy Scale | |
| | | | | Depression, anxiety, physical symptoms, illness worry | The Common Mental Disorders Questionnaire | |
| Pieber et al. [29] | 96 | 18 months | Multidisciplinary rehabilitation program. | Pain | Visual analog scale (VAS). | Persistent improvements in muscle strength, pain, function and quality of life in patients with chronic low back pain. |
| | | | | Physical disability | Roland–Morris disability Questionnaire (RM) | |
| | | | | Mobility | Range of motion (ROM) | |
| | | | | Muscle strength | Muscle strength | |
| | | | | Quality of life | Short Form Health Survey (SF-36) | |

| Reference | Sample | Follow-up time | Intervention | Measurement | Instrument | Outcomes |
|-----------|--------|----------------|--------------|-------------|------------|----------|
| Verkerk et al. [31] | 1.760 | 5 and 12 months | Multidisciplinary therapy | Pain | Visual analog scale (VAS) | 30% Improvement Between Baseline and 5- and 12-month follow-ups. |
| | | | | Fatigue | Fegree of present fatigue | The prognostic factors were: being married or living with one adult, |
| | | | | Kinesiophobia | Tampa Scale for Kinesiophobia (TSK) score | having no comorbidity, younger age, a higher education level, higher disability score at baseline, |
| | | | | Quality of life | Short Form Health Survey (SF-36) | no previous rehabilitation, reporting low pain intensity at baseline, and a higher score on the SF-36 and PCS. |
| | | | | | Physical Component Summary (PCS) Mental Component Summary (MCS]) | |
| Koele et al. [32] | 165 | 21 months | 15-week multidisciplinary rehabilitation program | Pain | Numerical rating scale (NRS pain) | Improvements in pain, activities and participation over time. |
| | | | | Disability | Pain Disability Index (PDI) The Multidimensional Pain Inventory (MPI) | |
| | | | | Pain catastrophizing | Pain Catastrophizing Scale (PCS) | |
| | | | | Fatigue | Numerical rating scale (NRS fatigue) | |
| | | | | Overall quality of life | Short Form Health Survey (SF-36) | |
| Pietilä Holmner et al. [33] | 93 | 8 years | Interdisciplinary team assessment and a 4-week rehabilitation program | Pain | Visual analog scale (VAS) The Multidimensional Pain Inventory (MPI) | There were significant differences seen in pain severity, interference of daily living, life control, negative mood, support, as well as anxiety and depression. |
| | | | | Anxiety, depression | Hospital Anxiety and Depression Scale | |

| Reference | Sample | Follow-up time | Intervention | Measurement | Instrument | Outcomes |
|---|---|---|---|---|---|---|
| Gerdle et al. [30] | 227 | 12 months | Multimodal rehabilitation programs (MMRP) | Characteristics of pain | Numeric rating scale | There were strong improvements in pain intensity and emotional aspect. |
| | | | | | Multidimensional Pain Inventory (MPI) | |
| | | | | | | The significant predictors were weak. |
| | | | | | Hospital Anxiety and Depression Scale (HADS) | |
| | | | | | The Chronic Pain Acceptance Questionnaire (CPAQ) | |
| | | | | | The Tampa Scale for Kinesiophobia Life Satisfaction Questionnaire (LISAT-11) | |
| | | | | | The Short Form Health Survey (SF36) | |
| Gardner et al. [34] | 20 392 | 2 months | Test the preliminar effectiveness of a patient-led goal-setting intervention | Disability | The European Quality of Life instrument (EQ-5D) The Quebec Back Pain Disability Scale (QBPDS) | Disability, pain intensity, physical quality of life, mental quality of life, total quality of life, self-efficacy and fear avoidance measures improved significantly between baseline and 2 months. |
| | | | | Pain intensity | Numerical rating scale (NRS pain) | Non-significant changes occurred in depression, anxiety and stress (P = 0.78). |
| | | | | Quality of life | Short Form Health Survey (SF-36) | |
| | | | | Negative emotional states of depression, anxiety and stress | The Depression Anxiety Stress Scale (DASS) | |
| | | | | Self-efficacy | Pain Self-Efficacy Questionnaire (PSEQ) | |
| | | | | Fear of movement/ (re) injury | Tampa Scale for Kinesiophobia (TSK) | |

| Reference | Sample | Follow-up time | Intervention | Measurement | Instrument | Outcomes |
|---|---|---|---|---|---|---|
| Jensen et al. [28] | | 3.5 years | Pain acceptance | Pain acceptance | Chronic Pain Acceptance Questionnaire (CPAQ) | In every case, higher initial levels of pain acceptance were associated with better outcomes over time; ie, more improvement in depressive symptoms and sleep disturbance, and less increase in pain intensity and pain interference.<br><br>Positive and significant association between change in pain and change in depression among those with relatively low activity engagement acceptance |
| | | | | Average pain intensity | | |
| | | | | Pain interference | Numerical rating scale (NRS pain) | |
| | | | | Deppresive symptoms | Patient-Reported Outcomes Measurement | |
| | | | | Physical function | Information System (PROMIS) | |
| | | | | Sleep disturbance | | |

**Table 2.** Therapeutic approaches for chronic musculoskeletal pain.

interference of pain in activities, in physical function, depressive symptoms and quality of sleep, which manage to endure over time [28].

When the intervention of chronic lower back pain is based on multidisciplinary rehabilitation including sensorimotor training, aerobic resistance, education and stress management, significant improvements were observed on lumbar extensor strength, range of motion, pain intensity and quality of life. These improvements persisted long term, over 18 months after the intervention had ceased [29].

A 12-month monitoring of a multimodal chronic pain rehabilitation programme reported significant improvements regarding pain, psychological symptoms, social participation, health and quality of life, although this type of approach requires more research support [30].

The observation of a 2-month multidisciplinary approach (16 sessions) in 1760 patients with lower back pain showed a greater than 30% reduction in disability after a follow-up of 5 and 12 months after the intervention, recognizing influential prognostic factors among the controlled patients, such as improved self-perception of health, a lower degree of initial disability, no co-morbidities and a positive prognosis relation at a younger age [31].

Predictors of the improved results of multidisciplinary therapy as regards to generalized pain are associated with greater self-efficacy, lower anxiety, higher educational levels, less beliefs about the consequences and the male sex. Therefore, this information indicates that we should guide treatment towards these specific characteristics and/or facilitate the selection of patients that will have a better response to this type of treatment based on this information [32].

An interdisciplinary evaluation performed over 8 years after a 4 week rehabilitation programme in 93 women with chronic musculoskeletal pain, showed a significant short-term and long-term improvement in pain, control of anxiety and depression [33].

Additionally, a novel pilot study based on a therapeutic approach with the establishment of objectives led by the patients themselves and supervised by a physiotherapist specialized in chronic lower back pain, showed significant improvements on quality of life, pain intensity, self-efficacy, fear-avoidance and level of disability, after 2 months of intervention and after a 2 month follow-up. This supports the importance of therapeutic goals being based on the patient when planning an intervention plan [34]. Another study reported that including the distraction of pain in the therapeutic process benefited patients with chronic pain, especially those who show greater catastrophism. Therefore, the increase in pain intensity could be due to a higher level of attention to pain (hypervilance) [35] (**Figure 1**).

In conclusion, this review about the evidence from existing cohort studies related to chronic musculoskeletal pain oriented on the understanding of risk factors, prognostic factors, protective factors and therapeutic approaches, allows us to extract important information for recognizing different clinical and psychosocial components involved in this condition that generally affect patients. This helps us to understand the characteristics of their behaviour and the pertinent therapeutic projections; facilitating the development of good clinical practices.

Although it is true that observational research regarding chronic musculoskeletal pain remains insufficient, there is still some important information that potentiates our understanding and redirects the rehabilitation of chronic pain; emphasizing the contribution of existing and related controlled clinical trials, proposing a rehabilitation programme based on biopsychosocial care, trying to cover all the involved factors and dimensions, and giving way to polymodal and interdisciplinary intervention.

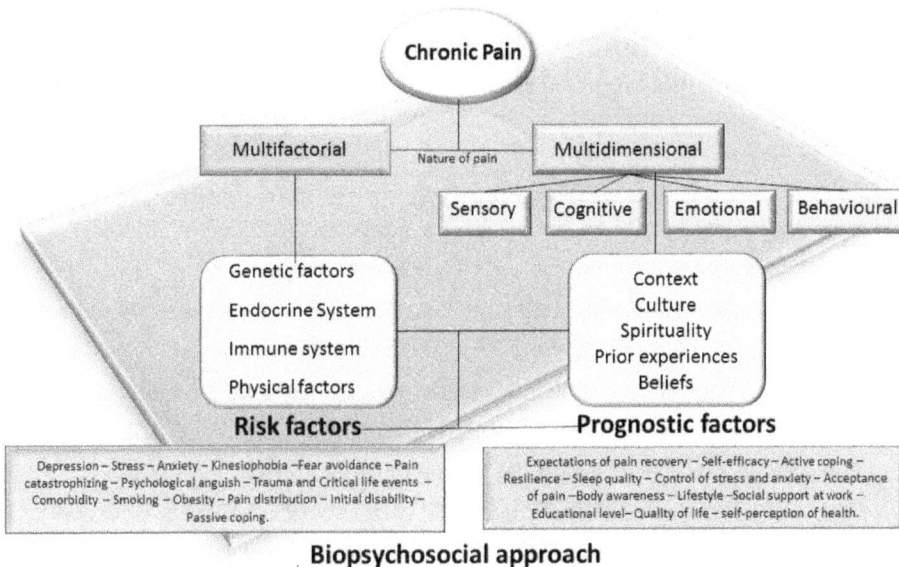

**Figure 1.** Conceptual model of chronic pain.

The contribution of cohort studies to the understanding of chronic musculoskeletal pain, is supported under the methodological rigor of objectively establishing the definition of results of the observed variables, and favors the control of biases by using different instruments to obtain measurements that allow a conclusive description of an outcome. In the case of the assessment of pain intensity, the studies reviewed used the visual analogue scale (VAS), the McGill pain questionnaire, scale for the numerical assessment of pain, and the pain inventory. Regarding exposure variables for psychosocial factors such as pain catastrophizing, self-perception of health, stress, anxiety, perception of disability, etc., the studies applied the catastrophizing scale of pain, Tampa scale of kinesiophobia, arthritis self-efficacy scale, the common mental disorders questionnaire, the quality of life survey (SF-36), the pain disability index, and the Roland–Morris disability questionnaire, among others.

## Author details

Cristhian Saavedra Santiesteban

Address all correspondence to: cristhian.saavedra@uach.cl

School of Kinesiology, Universidad Austral de Chile, Valdivia, Chile

## References

[1]  Henschke N, Kamper S, Maher C. The epidemiology and economic consequences of pain. Mayo Clinic Proceedings. 2015, Jan;90(1):139-147. DOI:10.1016/j.mayocp.2014.09.010

[2]  Reid KJ, Harker J, Bala MM. Epidemiology of chronic non-cancer pain in Europe: Narrative review of prevalence, pain treatments and pain impact. Current Medical Research and Opinion. 2011, Feb;27(2):449-462. DOI: 10.1185/03007995.2010.545813

[3]  Geurts J, Willems P, Lockwood C. Patient expectations for management of chronic non-cancer pain: A systematic review. Health Expectations. 2017, Dec;20(6):1201-1217. DOI: 10.1111/hex.12527

[4]  Carr D. Pain is a public health problem — What does that mean and why should we care? Pain Medicine. 2016;17:626-627. DOI: 10.1093/pm/pnw045

[5]  International Association for the Study of Pain. IASP Taxonomy [Internet]. 2018. Available from: https://www.iasp-pain.org/Taxonomy [Accessed: 08-11-2017]

[6]  van Hecke O, Torrance N, Smith BH. Chronic pain epidemiology and its clinical relevance. British Journal of Anaesthesia. 2013, Jul;111(1):13-18. DOI:10.1093/bja/aet123

[7]  Gaskin DJ, Richard P. The economic costs of pain in the United States. Pain. 2012, Aug;13(8): 715-724. DOI: 10.1016/j.jpain.2012.03.009

[8] Johannes CB, Le TK, Zhou X. The prevalence of chronic pain in United States adults: Results of an internet-based survey. The Journal of Pain. 2010, Nov;**11**(11):1230-1239. DOI: 10.1016/j.jpain.2010.07.002

[9] Blyth FM, March LM, Brnabic AJ. Chronic pain in Australia: A prevalence study. Pain. 2001, Jan;**89**(2-3):127-134

[10] Ibañez J. Situación actual del tratamiento del dolor crónico en España. Revista Española de Anestesiología y Reanimación. 2005;**52**:127-130

[11] Ospina M, Harstall C. Prevalence of chronic pain: An overview. Alberta Heritage Foundation for Medical Research. Edmonton, AB: Health Technology Assessment; 2002. Report N°28

[12] Catalá E, Reig E, Artés M. Prevalence of pain in the Spanish population: Telephone survey in 5000 homes. European Journal of Pain. 2002;**6**(2):133-140. DOI: 10.1053/eujp.2001.0310

[13] Larsson C, Hansson EE, Sundquist K. Chronic pain in older adults: Prevalence, incidence, and risk factors. Scandinavian Journal of Rheumatology. 2017, Jul;**46**(4):317-325. DOI: 10.1080/03009742.2016.1218543

[14] King S, Chambers CT, Huguet A. The epidemiology of chronic pain in children and adolescents revisited: A systematic review. Pain. 2011, Dec;**152**(12):2729-2738. DOI: 10.1016/j.pain.2011.07.016

[15] Engbers LH, Vollenbroek-Hutten MM, Van Harten WH. A comparison of patient characteristics and rehabilitation treatment content of chronic low back pain (CLBP) and stroke patients across six European countries. Health Policy. 2005, Mar;**71**(3):359-373. DOI: 10.1016/j.healthpol.2004.03.006

[16] Schofield DJ, Shrestha RN, Passey ME. Chronic disease and labour force participation among older Australians. The Medical Journal of Australia. 2008, Oct 20;**189**(8): 447-450

[17] Sleed M, Eccleston C, Beecham J. The economic impact of chronic pain in adolescence: Methodological considerations and a preliminary costs-of-illness study. Pain. 2005, Dec 15;**119**(1-3):183-190. DOI: 10.1016/j.pain.2005.09.028

[18] Phillips C. Economic burden of chronic pain. Expert Review of Pharmacoeconomics & Outcomes Research. 2006 Oct;**6**(5):591-601. DOI: 10.1586/14737167.6.5.591

[19] Fredrika KF, Lee DM, McBeth J. Chronic widespread pain is associated with worsening frailty in European men. Age and Ageing. 2016, Mar;**45**(2):274-280. DOI: 10.1093/ageing/afv170

[20] Andersen L, Clausen T, Persson R. Perceived physical exertion during healthcare work and prognosis for recovery from long-term pain in different body regions: Prospective cohort study. BMC Musculoskeletal Disorders. 2012;**13**:253. DOI: 10.1186/1471-2474-13-253

[21] Andersson H, Leden I. Serum uric acid predicts changes in reports of non-gouty chronic pain: A prospective study among women with inflammatory and non-inflammatory pain. Rheumatology International. 2012;**32**:193-198. DOI: 10.1007/s00296-010-1600-5

[22] Mehlsen M, Heegaard L, Frostholm L. A prospective evaluation of the chronic pain self-management Programme in a Danish population of chronic pain patients. Patient Education and Counseling. 2015, May;**98**(5):677-680. DOI: 10.1016/j.pec.2015.01.008

[23] Fuss I, Angst F, Lehmann S. Prognostic factors for pain relief and functional improvement in chronic pain after inpatient rehabilitation. The Clinical Journal of Pain. 2014, Apr;**30**(4): 279-285. DOI: 10.1097/AJP.0b013e31829a4d11

[24] Melloh M, Elfering A, Stanton TR. Who is likely to develop persistent low back pain? A longitudinal analysis of prognostic occupational factors. Work. 2013, Jan 1;**46**(3):297-311. DOI: 10.3233/WOR-131672

[25] Bohman T, Alfredsson L, Jensen I. Does a healthy lifestyle behaviour influence the prognosis of low back pain among men and women in a general population? A population-based cohort study. BMJ Open. 2014;**4**(12):e005713. DOI: 10.1136/bmjopen-2014-005713

[26] Williamson E, Williams M, Gates S. Risk factors for chronic disability in a cohort of patients with acute whiplash associated disorders seeking physiotherapy treatment for persisting symptoms. Physiotherapy. 2015;**101**:34-43. DOI: 10.1016/j.physio.2014.04.004

[27] Lundberg G, Gerdle B. The relationships between pain, disability, and health-related quality of life: An 8-year follow-up study of female home care personnel. Disability and Rehabilitation. 2016;**38**(3):235-244. DOI: 10.3109/09638288.2015.1035459

[28] Jensen M, Smith A, Alschuler K. The role of pain acceptance on function in individuals with disabilities: A longitudinal study. Pain. 2016, Jan;**157**(1):247-254. DOI: 10.1097/j.pain.0000000000000361

[29] Pieber K, Herceg M, Quittan M. Long-term effects of an outpatient rehabilitation program in patients with chronic recurrent low back pain. European Spine Journal. 2014;**23**:779-785. DOI: 10.1007/s00586-013-3156-z

[30] Gerdle B, Molander P, Stenberg G. Weak outcome predictors of multimodal rehabilitation at one-year follow-up in patients with chronic pain—A practice based evidence study from two SQRP centres. BMC Musculoskeletal Disorders. 2016;**17**:490. DOI: 10.1186/s12891-016-1346-7

[31] Verkerk K, Luijsterburg PA, Heymans MW. Prognosis and course of disability in patients with chronic nonspecific low back pain: A 5- and 12-month follow-up cohort study. Physical Therapy. 2013;**93**:1603-1614. DOI: 10.2522/ptj.20130076

[32] Koele R, Volker G, van Vree F. Multidisciplinary rehabilitation for chronic widespread musculoskeletal pain: Results from daily practice. Musculoskeletal Care. 2014, Dec;**12**(4): 210-220. DOI:10.1002/msc.1076

[33] Pietilä Holmner E, Fahlström M, Nordström A. The effects of interdisciplinary team assessment and a rehabilitation program for patients with chronic pain. Jan. 2013;**92**(1): 77-83. DOI: 10.1097/PHM.0b013e318278b28e

[34] Gardner T, Refshauge K. Patient led goal setting—A pilot study investigating a promising approach for the management of chronic low back pain. Spine (Phila Pa 1976). 2016, Sep 15;**41**(18):1405-1413. DOI: 10.1097/BRS.0000000000001545

[35] Schreiber KL, Campbell C, Martel MO. Distraction analgesia in chronic pain patients: The impact of catastrophizing. Anesthesiology. 2014, Dec;**121**(6):1292-1301. DOI: 10.1097/ ALN.0000000000000465

www.ingramcontent.com/pod-product-compliance
Lightning Source LLC
Chambersburg PA
CBHW081244190326
41458CB00016B/5913